INSTANT

Make-up

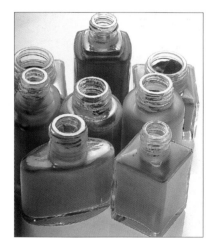

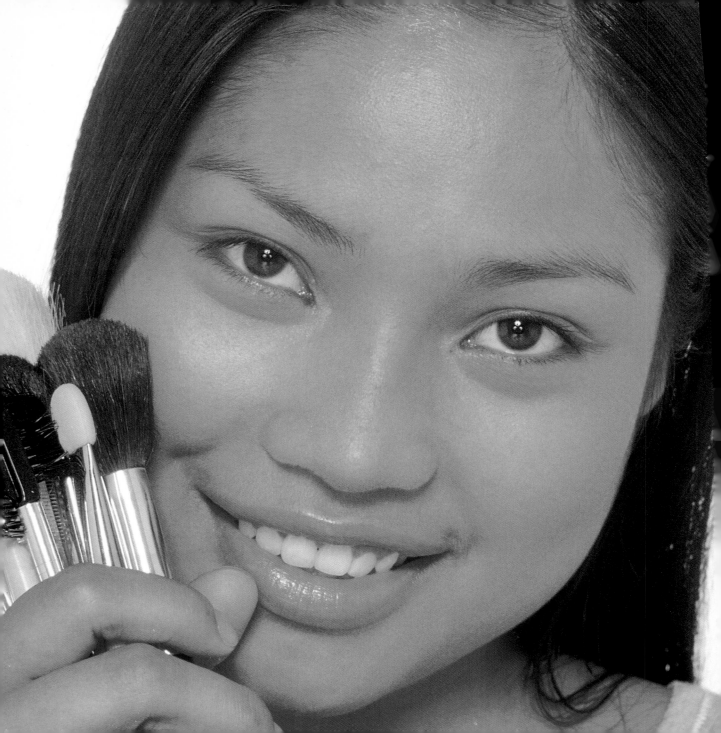

INSTANT
Make-up

The complete guide to looking good

Sally Norton

Photography: Nick Cole

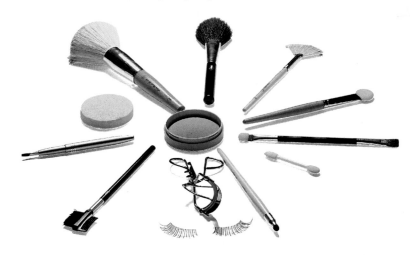

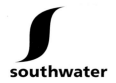

southwater

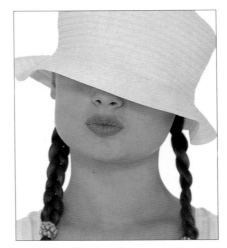

This edition is published by Southwater

Distributed in the UK by
The Manning Partnership
251–253 London Road East
Batheaston
Bath BA1 7RL
UK
tel. (0044) 01225 852 727
fax (0044) 01225 852 852

Distributed in Australia by
Sandstone Publishing
Unit 1, 360 Norton Street
Leichhardt
New South Wales 2040
Australia
tel. (0061) 2 9560 7888
fax (0061) 2 9560 7488

Distributed in New Zealand by
Five Mile Press NZ
PO Box 33-1071
Takapuna
Auckland 9
New Zealand
tel. (0064) 9 4444 144
fax (0064) 9 4444 518

Southwater is an imprint of Anness Publishing Limited
© 1998, 2000 Anness Publishing Limited

1 3 5 7 9 10 8 6 4 2

Publisher: Joanna Lorenz
Editor: Sarah Ainley
Designer: Siân Keogh, Axis Design
Photography: Nick Cole
Make-up & Hair: Debbi Finlow

Previously published as *Instant Make-up*

Contents

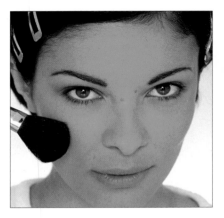 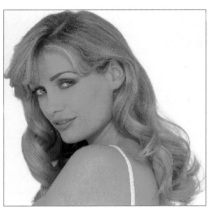 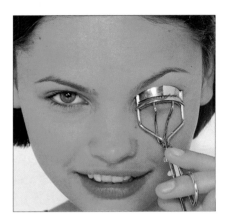

Make-up Magic

The key to making-up successfully is to understand how to enhance your features, using the best cosmetic formulations and colours around. This doesn't mean spending a small fortune on the latest season's colours and promotions. Instead, it means analyzing what will work for you, your colouring and your lifestyle, then making your purchases. If you wise up on the best of the products, brush up your application techniques and give yourself time to experiment, you can find the perfect look for you. And, once you've mastered the basics, you can solve your own particular beauty problems, and try out some inspirational make-up ideas – just for fun!

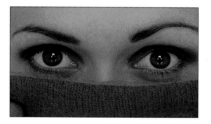

Above: Every woman can use make-up to emphasize her best features.

Right: Experiment with different styles to find the look that's right for you.

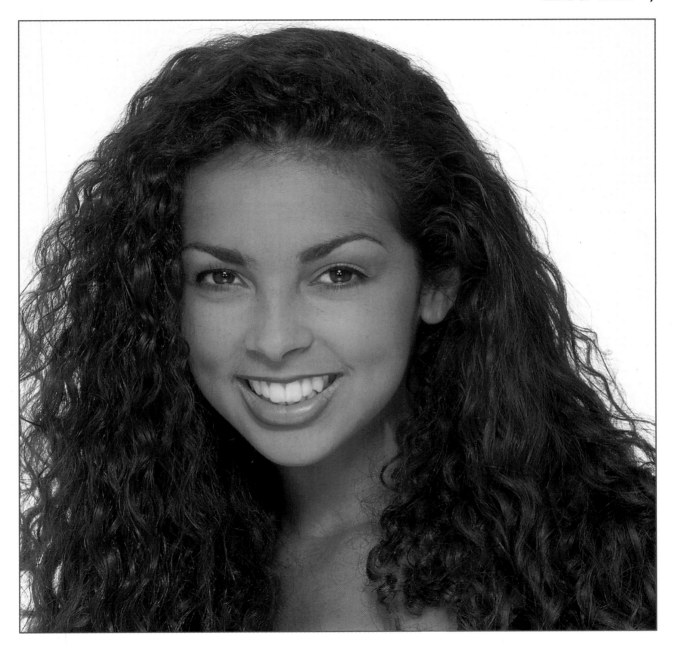

Eating for Beautiful Skin

While lotions and potions can improve your skin from the outside, a healthy diet works from the inside. A nutritious, balanced diet isn't only a delicious way to eat – it can work wonders for your skin.

YOU ARE WHAT YOU EAT

A diet for a healthy, clear complexion is the same one as for a healthy body. That is, one that contains lots of fresh fruit and vegetables, is high in fibre, low in fat, and low in added sugar and salt. This should provide your body and your skin with all the vitamins and minerals needed to function at their very best.

Healthy skin checklist

These are the essentials your body needs to keep your skin in tip-top condition.

1 The most essential element is water. Although there's water in the foods you eat, you should drink at least two litres (quarts) of water a day to keep your body healthy and your skin clear.

2 Cellulose carbohydrates, better known as fibre foods, have another less direct effect on the skin. Their action in keeping you regular can help to give you a brighter, clearer complexion.

3 Vitamin A is essential for growth and repair of certain skin tissues. Lack of it causes dryness, itching and loss of skin elasticity. It is found in foods such as carrots, spinach, broccoli and apricots.

4 Vitamin C is needed for collagen production, to help keep your skin firm and supple. It is found in foods such as strawberries, citrus fruits, cabbage, tomatoes and watercress.

5 Vitamin E is an antioxidant vitamin that neutralizes free radicals — highly reactive molecules that can cause ageing. It occurs in foods such as almonds, hazelnuts and wheat germ.

6 Zinc works with vitamin A in the making of collagen and elastin, the fibres that give your skin its strength, elasticity and firmness.

A healthy diet and a beautiful complexion go hand in hand. Eating too much and becoming overweight thickens the layer of fat under your skin and consequently stretches it. Crash dieting can then result in your skin collapsing, leading to the appearance of lines and wrinkles. What's more, a crash diet will deprive your skin and body of the essential nutrients they need to stay healthy and look good. If you need to lose weight, do it slowly, sensibly and steadily, to give your skin time to adjust. It is always advisable to consult your doctor before starting any weight loss programme.

A healthy low-fat, high-fibre diet is known to be good for skin so keep snacks such as chocolate to a minimum and eat them only as an occasional treat.

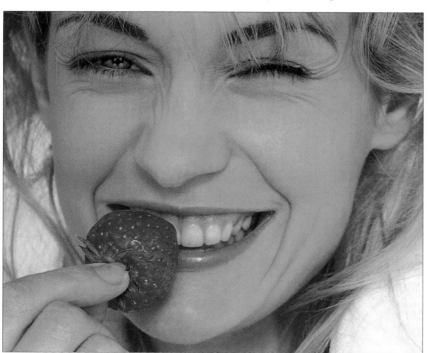

Left: Swap sugar-rich snacks for fresh fruit – it's a delicious way to give your skin a healthy boost.

Here's a good typical day's diet for a clearer complexion.

Breakfast: A glass of unsweetened fruit juice; bowl of unsweetened muesli (whole grain cereal), topped with a chopped banana and semi-skimmed (1 per cent or skim) milk. Two slices of whole wheat toast with a scraping of low-fat spread.

Lunch: Baked potato, filled with low-fat cottage cheese and plenty of fresh, raw salad. One low-fat yogurt, any flavour.

Evening meal: Grilled (broiled) fish or chicken, with boiled brown rice, and steamed vegetables. Fresh fruit salad, topped with natural yogurt and chopped nuts.

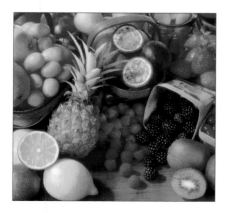

Above: Beautiful skin, like a healthy body, needs plenty of fresh fruit and vegetables to keep it radiant and supple.

Right: It's clearly obvious that drinking plenty of water during the day helps purify your body – which means a fresher, firmer skin.

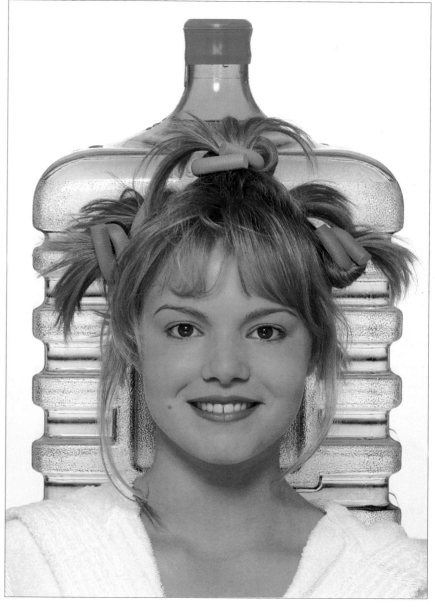

A Fabulous Foundation

Many women avoid wearing foundation because they're scared of an unnatural, mask-like effect. In fact, finding the right product for you is simpler than you might think. There are two keys to success: the first is to choose the perfect shade and the second is to pick the right formulation for your skin. With this shade and formulation selection, you can get the best coverage for your particular skin-type.

Tinted moisturizers

These are a cross between a moisturizer and a foundation, as they'll soothe your skin while giving a little coverage. They're ideal for young or clear skins. They're also great in the summer, when you want a sheer effect or to even out a fading tan. Unlike other foundations, you can blend tinted moisturizers on with your fingertips.

Liquid foundations

These suit all but the driest skins. If you have oily skin or suffer from breakouts, look for an oil-free liquid foundation to cover affected areas without aggravating them.

Cream foundations

These are thick, rich and moisturizing, making them ideal for dry or mature skins. They have a fairly heavy texture, so blend them well into your skin with a damp cosmetic sponge.

Mousse foundations

Again these are quite moisturizing, and ideal for drier skins. To apply, dab a little onto the back of your hand, then dot onto your skin with a sponge.

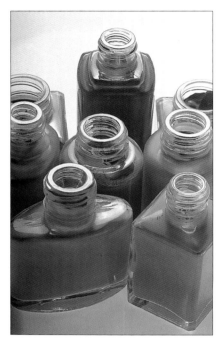

Above: Choose from a range of shades.

Compact foundations

These are all-in-one formulations, which already contain powder. They come in a compact, usually with their own sponge for application. They actually give a lighter finish than you'd expect.

Stick foundations

These are the original foundation, dating back to the early days of Hollywood. They have a heavy texture and so are best confined for use on badly blemished or scarred skin. Dot a little foundation directly onto the affected area, then blend gently with a damp sponge.

SHADE SELECTION

Once you've chosen the ideal formulation for you, you're ready to choose the perfect shade to match your skin.

■ Ensure you're in natural daylight when trying out foundation colours, so you can see exactly how your skin will look once you leave the shop or counter.

■ Select a couple of shades to try, which look as though they'll match your skin.

■ Don't try foundation on your hand or on your wrist – they're a different colour than your face.

■ Stroke a little colour onto your jawline to ensure you get a tone that will blend with your neck as well as your face. The shade that seems to "disappear" into your skin is the right one for you.

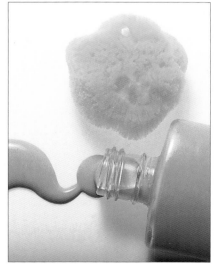

Above: Liquid foundation.

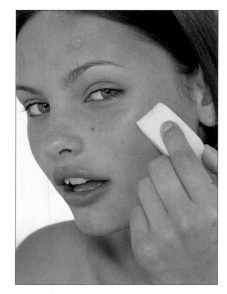

Above: Blend, blend, blend for a professional finish. And don't forget to give your face a final check to make sure you haven't got any unnatural lines where your foundation finishes.

APPLICATION KNOW-HOW

■ Apply foundation to freshly-moisturized skin to ensure you have a perfect base on which to work.

■ Use a cosmetic sponge to apply most types of foundation – using your fingertips can result in an uneven, greasy finish.

■ Apply foundation in dots, then blend each one with your sponge.

■ Dampen the sponge first of all, then squeeze out the excess moisture – this will prevent the sponge from soaking up too much costly foundation.

■ Check for "tidemarks" (streaks) on your jawline, nose, forehead and chin.

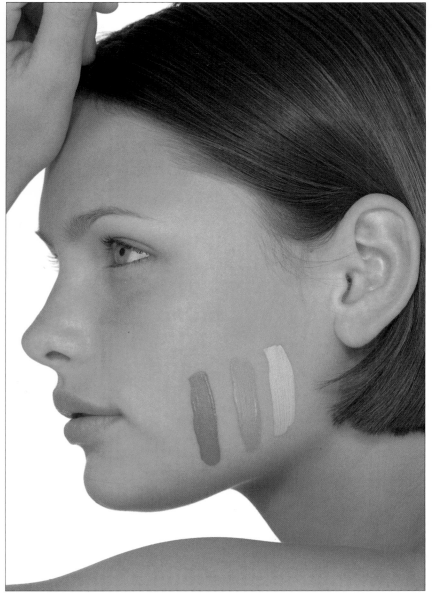

Above: Check different foundation colours on your jawline for the perfect match.

The Cover Up

Concealers are a fast and effective way to disguise blemishes, so your skin looks perfect. They're a concentrated form of foundation with a very high pigment content, so they offer complete coverage to problem areas. Applying them after foundation is best, as they are only applied to specific areas, and these would be disturbed if foundation is applied over the top.

Stick concealers

These are easy to apply as you can simply stroke them straight onto the skin. They're the most readily available type on the market. Some have quite a heavy and thick consistency, so it's worth trying out the different samples in the shop before you buy.

Cream concealers

These usually come in a tube, with a sponge-tipped applicator. The coverage isn't as thick as the stick type, but the finished effect is very natural.

Liquid concealers

Again, these come in a tube. Just squeeze a tiny amount of product onto your finger and smooth over the affected area. Look for the cream-to-powder formulations, which slick on like a cream and dry to a velvety powder finish.

> ### Concealer Tip
> When choosing a concealer look for the colour nearest to your own skin-tone rather than a lighter one. Covering a problem area with a paler shade will simply accentuate it.

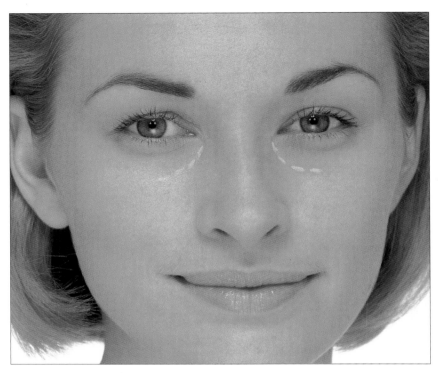

TAKING COVER

Here's how to conceal all your beauty problems effectively.

Spots and blemishes

The ideal solution is to use a medicated stick concealer as these contain ingredients to deal with the pimple or blemish as well as cover it. Only apply the concealer exactly on the pimple or blemish, as they can be quite drying, and then smooth away the edges with a clean cotton bud (swab). Applying concealer all around the area will make the spot more noticeable and create a "halo" effect.

Above: Hide under-eye shadows with a few dots of concealer. If you're after a light make-up effect, apply concealer directly onto clean skin, then apply powder or all-in-one foundation/ powder over the top.

Under-eye shadows

Opt for a creamy stick concealer or a liquid one, as dry formulations will emphasize fine lines around your eyes. If you're blending with your fingertips, use your ring finger, as this is the weakest finger on your hand and less likely to drag at the delicate skin.

Pow! Wow! Powder!

Face powder is the make-up artist's best friend, as it can make your skin look really wonderful and is very versatile in its uses. Choose one that closely matches your skin-tone for a natural effect. Do this by dusting a little on your jawline, in the same way as you would with foundation.

■ Powder gives a super-smooth sheen to your skin – with or without foundation.

■ It "sets" your foundation, so it stays put and looks good for longer.

■ Powder absorbs oils from your skin, and helps prevent shiny patches.

■ It helps conceal open pores.

Loose powder

This gives the best and longest-lasting finish and is the choice of professional make-up artists and models. The best way to apply loose powder is to dust it lightly onto your skin using a large, soft powder brush. Then brush over your face again lightly to dust off the excess.

Pressed powder

Most come with their own application sponges, but you'll find you get a better result if you apply them with a brush. Look for brushes with retractable heads.

If you do use the sponge, use a light touch, and wash it regularly, or you'll transfer the oils in your skin onto the powder and get a build-up.

Above Right: Powder gives a perfect featherlight finish to your skin.

Right: Choose the shade that best suits your skin colouring.

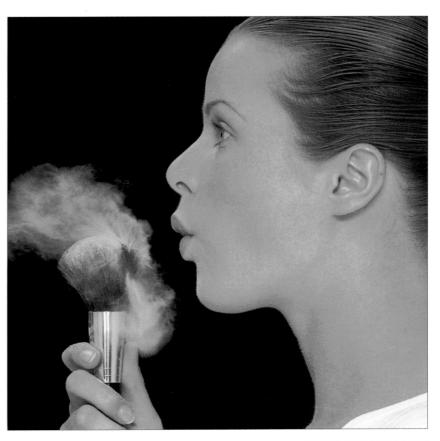

Powder Tip

When dusting excess powder away from your skin, use your brush in light, downward strokes to help prevent the powder from getting caught in the fine hairs on your skin. Pay particular attention to the sides of the face and jawline which aren't so easy for you to see.

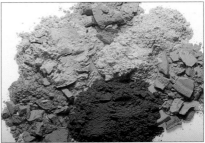

Blush Baby

Give your complexion a bloom of colour with this indispensable beauty aid.

Powder blusher

This should be applied over the top of your foundation and face powder. To apply powder blusher, dust over the compact with a large soft brush. If you've taken too much onto your brush, tap the handle on the back of your hand to remove the excess. It's better to waste a little blusher than apply too much!

Start the colour on the fullest parts of your cheeks, directly below the centre of your eyes. Then smile and dust the blusher over your cheekbones, and up towards your temples. Blend the colour well towards the hairline, so you avoid harsh edges. This will place colour where you would naturally blush.

Right: Brush your cheeks with colour.

Below: Be a blushing beauty with a light touch of powder blusher.

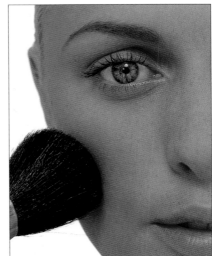

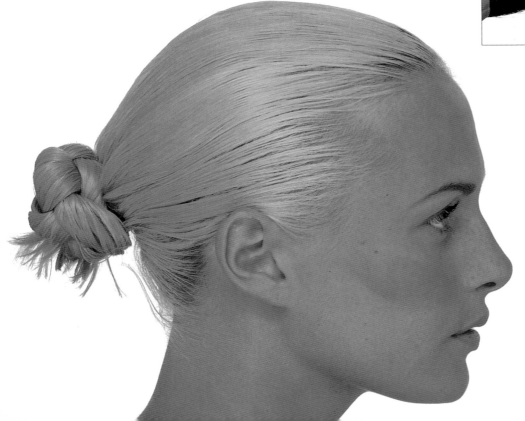

Cream blusher

Cream blusher is applied with your fingertips, after foundation, but before face powder. To apply, dab a few dots over your cheeks, from the plump part up towards your cheekbone. Using your fingertips, blend well. Build up the effect gradually, adding more blusher to create just the look you want. Or, if you prefer, you can use a foundation wedge to blend in cream blusher.

Colour choice

There's always a kaleidoscope of blusher shades to choose from. However, as a general rule, it's best to opt for a shade that tones well with your skin colouring, and co-ordinates with the rest of your make-up. You can opt for lighter or darker shades, depending on the season.

COLOUR GUIDE

Colouring	Choose
Blonde hair, cool skin	Pale pink shades
Blonde hair, warm skin	Pinky-brown shades
Dark hair, cool skin	Rose-pink shades
Dark hair, warm skin	Rose-brown shades
Red hair, cool skin	Pale peach shades
Red hair, warm skin	Warm peach shades
Dark hair, olive skin	Warm brown shades
Black hair, dark skin	Brown-red shades

Right: Powder blusher is a quick and easy option.

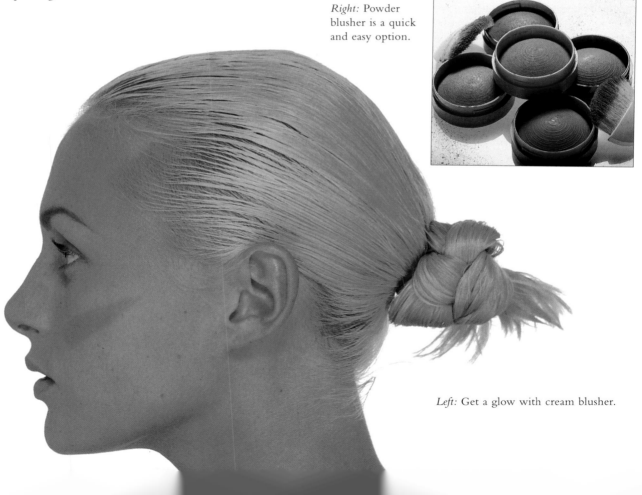

Left: Get a glow with cream blusher.

The Eyes Have It

Eye make-up is the most popular type of cosmetic, and for good reason. Just the simplest touch of mascara can open up your eyes, while a splash of colour can transform them instantly. Whatever your eye shape and colour, you can ensure that they always look beautiful.

EYEBROW KNOW-HOW

Many women overlook their eyebrows, or sometimes even worse, overpluck them. When it comes to eye make-up, the eyebrows make an important impression. They can provide a balanced look to your face so it's well worth making the effort to get them looking right.

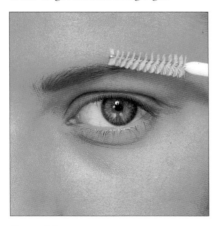

Natural brows
For perfectly groomed brows in an instant, try combing through them with a brush to flick away any powder or foundation. Comb the hairs upwards and outwards. This will also help give you a wide-eyed look. Then lightly slick them with clear gel to hold the shape neatly in place.

Eyebrow colour
To define your brows you can use eyebrow powder or pencil.

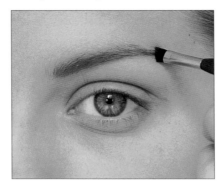

1 Apply powder with an eyebrow brush, dusting it through your brows and taking care not to sweep it onto the surrounding skin. This gives a natural effect, and requires little blending.

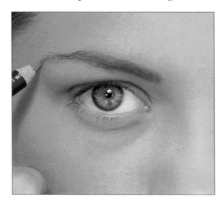

2 Alternatively, use a well-sharpened pencil to draw on tiny strokes, taking care not to press too hard or the finished effect will be unnatural.

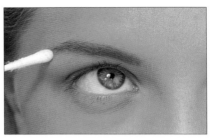

3 Then soften the lines you've made with the eye pencil by lightly stroking a clean cotton bud (swab) through your brows.

LINING UP LINER

Eyeliner is a great way to flatter all eye shapes and sizes. Eyeliner should be applied after eyeshadow and before your mascara.

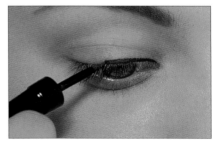

Liquid liners
These have a fluid consistency, and usually come with a brush attached to the cap. However, these aren't as easy to apply as the "ink-well" sponge-tipped variety. To apply the liner, look down into your mirror to prevent the liquid smudging. You should stay like this for a few seconds after applying the liner to give it time to dry thoroughly.

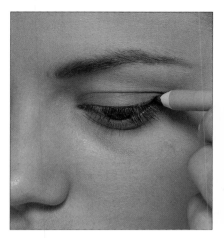

Pencil liners

This is the easiest way to add extra emphasis to your eyes. A pencil should be used to draw a line close to your upper and lower lashes. It's a good idea to sharpen the pencil between uses, not only to ensure you have a fine tip with which to work, but also to keep it bacteria-free.

Draw a soft line close to your lashes. If you find this quite difficult, try dotting it on along your lashes, then joining up the dots afterwards! Run over the pencil line with a brush. Alternatively, look for pencils that come with a smudger built in at the other end.

Eyeliner Know-How

If you've never applied liner before and feel a bit nervous, try this technique. Sit down at a table in a good light with a mirror. Take your eyeliner in your hand and rest your elbow on the table to keep your arm and hand steady. You can also give yourself extra support by resting your little finger on your cheek.

Eyeshadow as eyeliner

Make-up artists often use eyeshadow to outline the eyes, and it's a trick worth stealing! It looks great because it gives a very soft smoky effect.

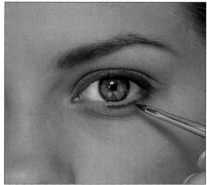

1 Use a small brush to apply shadow under your lower lashes and to make an impact over the top of the eyelid, taking care to keep the shadow close to the eyelashes.

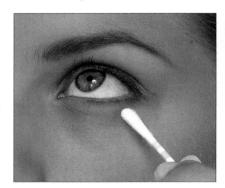

2 To create a softer, more modern effect simply sweep over the eyeshadow liner with a clean cotton bud (swab).

MASCARA MAGIC

Mascara adds a flattering fringe to your eyes – particularly if your lashes are fair.

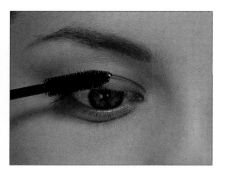

1 Start by applying mascara to your upper lashes first. Brush them downwards to start with, then brush your lashes upwards from underneath. Use a tiny zig-zag movement to prevent mascara from clogging on your lashes.

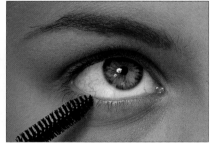

2 Next, use the tip of the mascara wand to brush your lower lashes, using a gentle side-to-side technique. Take care to keep your hand steady whilst you are applying the mascara, and not to blink whilst the mascara is still wet. Comb through your lashes with an eyelash comb to remove any excess the wand has left behind.

Below: Beautiful eyes – naturally.

Bottom Right: Experiment with different coloured powder shadows.

EYEING UP EYESHADOWS

Choose neutral colours to subtly enhance your looks, or play with a kaleidoscope of different shades to contrast with and dramatize your colouring.

Powder eyeshadows

The most popular type, these come in pressed cakes of powder either with a small brush or a sponge applicator. You can build up their density from barely-there to dramatic. Apply using a damp brush or sponge if you want a deep colour for an evening look.

Cream shadows

These are oil-based and come in little pots or compacts. They're applied either with a brush or your fingertips. They're a good choice for dry skins that need extra moisturizing.

Stick shadows

Wax-based, you smooth these onto your eyelids from the stick. Ensure they have a creamy texture before you buy them, so they won't drag at your skin.

Liquid shadows

Usually these come in a slim bottle with a sponge applicator. Look for the cream-to-powder ones that smooth on as a liquid and blend to a velvety powder finish.

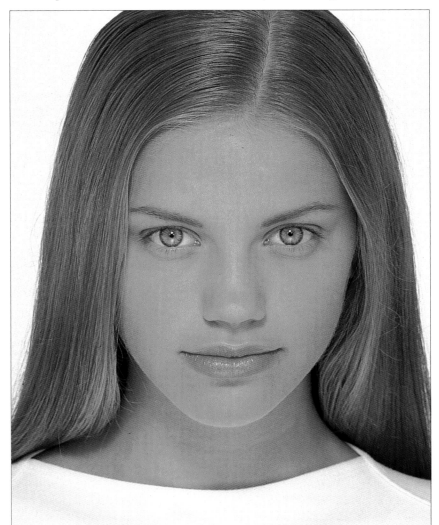

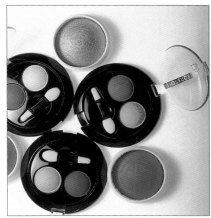

Brush Up Your Make-up

Even the most expensive make-up in the world won't look particularly great if it's applied carelessly and using your fingertips. For a professional finish you need the right tools. Here's your basic kit.

Make-up sponge

It is best to have a wedge-shaped make-up sponge, so you can use the finer edges to help blend in foundation round your nose and jawline, while the flatter edges are great for the cheeks, forehead and chin. However, if you prefer not to use a synthetic sponge you can try the small, natural ones instead.

Powder brush

Get used to using a powder brush each time you put make-up on. To prevent a caked or clogged finish to your face powder, use a large, soft brush to dust away any excess.

Blusher brush

Use to add a pretty glow to your skin with a light dusting of powder blusher. A blusher brush is slightly smaller than a powder brush to make it easier to control.

Eyeshadow brush

Smooth on any shade of eyeshadow with this brush.

Eyebrow tweezers

It is essential to have a good pair of tweezers for regularly tidying up the eyebrows.

Eyeshadow sponge

A sponge applicator is great for applying a sweep of pale eyeshadow that does not need much blending, or for applying highlighter to your brow bones.

All-in-one eyelash brush/comb

Great for combing through your lashes between coats of mascara for a clump-free finish. Flip the comb over and use the brush side to sweep your eyebrows into shape, or soften pencilled-in brows.

Lipbrush

Use to create a perfect outline for your lips and then use to fill in the shape with your lipstick.

Eyelash curlers

Once used, they'll soon become a beauty essential! Curlier eyelashes help open up your eyes and make a huge difference to the way you look.

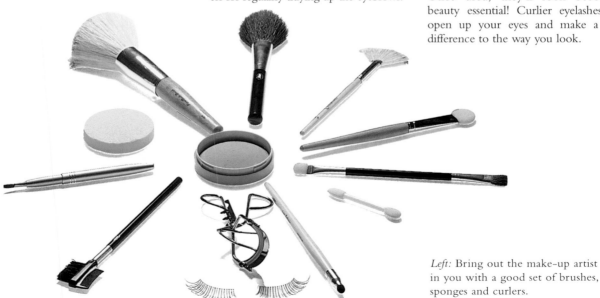

Left: Bring out the make-up artist in you with a good set of brushes, sponges and curlers.

Eye Make-up Masterclass

Now that you know where to start, you can experiment with more sophisticated eye make-up methods to create a variety of stunning looks. Here's a look you can try, using a wide range of techniques to create the ultimate in glamorous eye make-up.

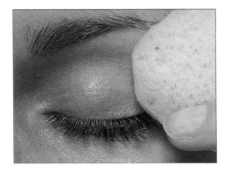

1 Smooth over your eyelids with foundation to create an even base on which to work, and to give your eye make-up something to cling to.

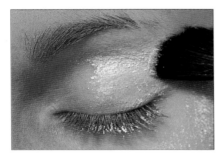

2 Sweep over your eyelids with a brush loaded with translucent face powder. Dust a little translucent powder under your eyes to catch any flecks of fallen eyeshadow later.

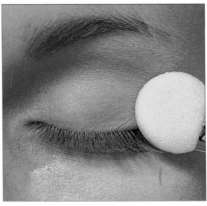

3 Use a sponge applicator to sweep a neutral ivory shade over your eyelids. Work it right up towards your eyebrows for a balanced overall effect.

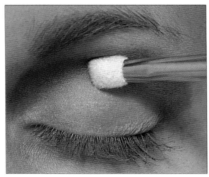

4 Smudge a brown eyeshadow into the socket line of your eyes, using a sponge applicator. If you find blending difficult, try using a slightly shimmery powder as these are easier to work in. Use a brush to sweep over the top of the brown shadow as this will remove any harsh edges.

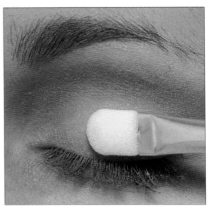

5 To create a perfectly blended finish, sweep some more ivory shadow over the edges of the brown eyeshadow using a sponge applicator. Now that you've completed your eyeshadow, flick away the powder from under your eyes.

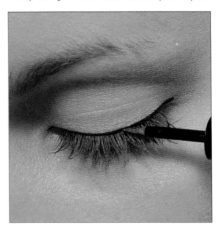

6 Looking down into a mirror and keeping your hand steady, apply liquid eyeliner along your upper lashes.

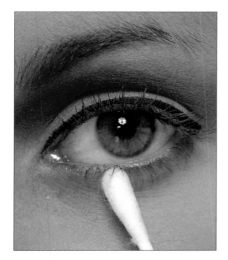

7 Use a clean cotton bud (swab) to work some brown eyeshadow under your lower lashes to add some subtle definition.

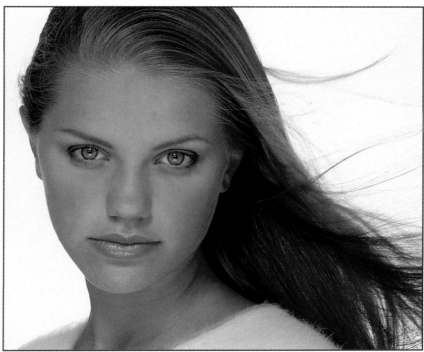

Above: For our main look here, we used a palette of ivory and blue eyeshadow, combined with black eyeliner and mascara. Take time to experiment with different colours to find a look that suits you and your colouring.

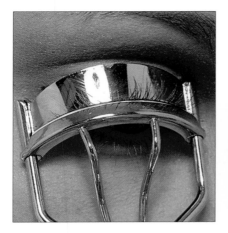

8 Squeeze your lashes with eyelash curlers to make them bend, before applying mascara. This will "open up" the eye area.

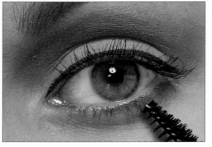

9 Apply mascara onto your upper lashes and use the tip of the mascara wand to coat your lower lashes.

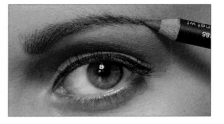

10 Stroke your eyebrows with pencil to shape them and fill in any patches. Smooth over the top with a cotton bud (swab) to soften the eyebrow pencil line.

Getting Lippy

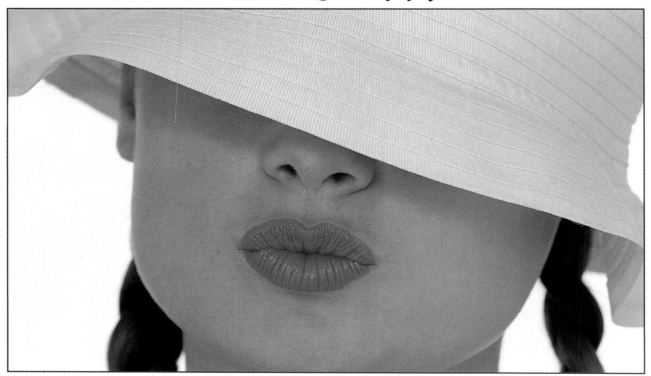

Lipstick has been around for about 5,000 years! It's the easiest and quickest way to give your face a focus and create an instant splash of colour.

A LICK OF COLOUR

■ Lipsticks in a bullet form are the most popular way to use lip colour. Some lipsticks even come with in-built Sun Protection sunscreens.

■ Another way of applying colour is with a lip gloss. These can be used alone to give your lips an attractive sheen, or over the top of lipstick to catch the light.

■ Lipliners are used to provide an outline to your lips before applying lipstick. You can also use them over your entire lip for a dark, matte effect. However, you may need to add a touch of lipsalve (balm) over the top to prevent drying out this delicate area of skin.

Above: A slick of colour will make you love your lips. The best way to apply lipstick is with a lipbrush.

Right: A selection of lipstick colours is the key to creating different looks.

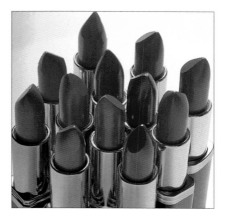

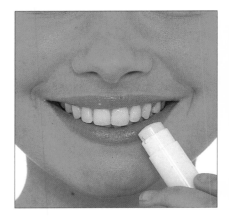

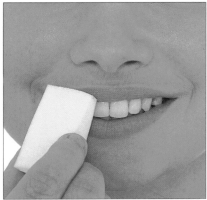

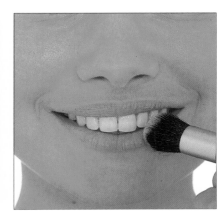

1 Ensure your lips are soft and supple by smoothing over moisturizer before you start.

2 Prime your lips by smoothing them with foundation, using a make-up sponge so you reach every tiny crevice on the surface.

3 Dust over the top of the foundation with a light dusting of your usual face powder, to help your lipstick stay put for longer.

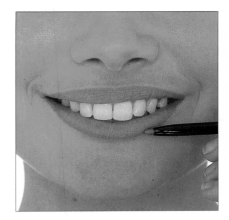

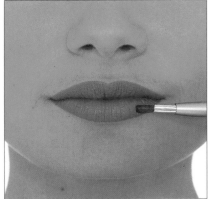

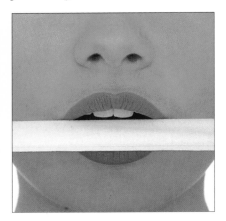

4 Rest your elbow on a firm surface and carefully draw an outline using a lip pencil. So it doesn't drag your skin, it may help to warm it slightly in your palm. Start by defining the Cupid's bow on the upper lip, then draw a neat outline on your lower lip. Finish by completing the edges of the outline to your upper lip.

5 Use a lipbrush to fill in the outline with lipstick, ensuring you reach into every tiny crevice on the surface. Open your mouth to brush the colour into the corners of your lips.

6 You'll help your lipstick last longer if you blot over the surface with a tissue. It'll also give an attractive, semi-matte finish to your lips. Reapply to help a longer-lasting finish.

Cool Skin, Blonde Hair

With your porcelain complexion and pale hair, you should opt for baby pastel tones with sheer formulations and a hint of shimmer. This way you'll flatter your colouring with a light, fresh make-up look, without overpowering it.

THIS LOOK SUITS YOU IF...

■ You have pale blonde to mousy or mid-blonde hair.

■ Your eyes are blue, grey, hazel or green.

■ You have pale skin, including whiter-than-white, ivory or a pinky "English rose" complexion.

Tip

If you're older, or unsure about wearing blue eyeshadow, swap it for a cool grey. This will create the same soft effect, but it's more subtle. You may prefer to switch to matte ivory instead of shimmery eyeshadow.

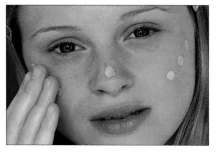

1 Your delicate skin doesn't need heavy coverage, so use a light tinted moisturizer. Dot it lightly onto your nose, cheeks, forehead and chin, then blend it in with your fingertips.

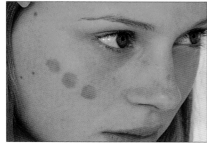

2 Cool pink blusher will give a soft glow to your skin. Dot onto your cheeks, then blend in with your fingertips. Either skip powder to leave your skin with a dewy glow, or gently dust a little over your face.

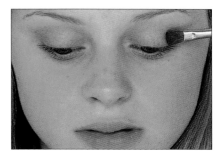

3 Take a baby blue eyeshadow onto an eyeshadow brush and sweep it evenly over your entire eyelid. Stroke the brush gently over your eyelid a few times until you've swept away any obvious edges to the eyeshadow.

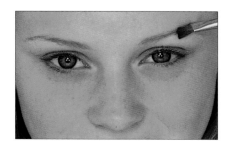

4 Sweep a shimmery ivory shadow from the crease in your eyelid up towards the brow bone to open up the eye area.

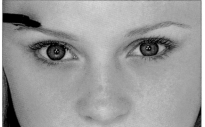

5 Stroke your eyebrow into shape with an eyebrow brush. This will also flick away any powder that's got caught in the hairs.

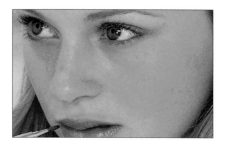

6 Cool pink lipstick should be applied with a lipbrush. If you like, you can slick a little lipgloss or lip balm on top for a sexy shimmer.

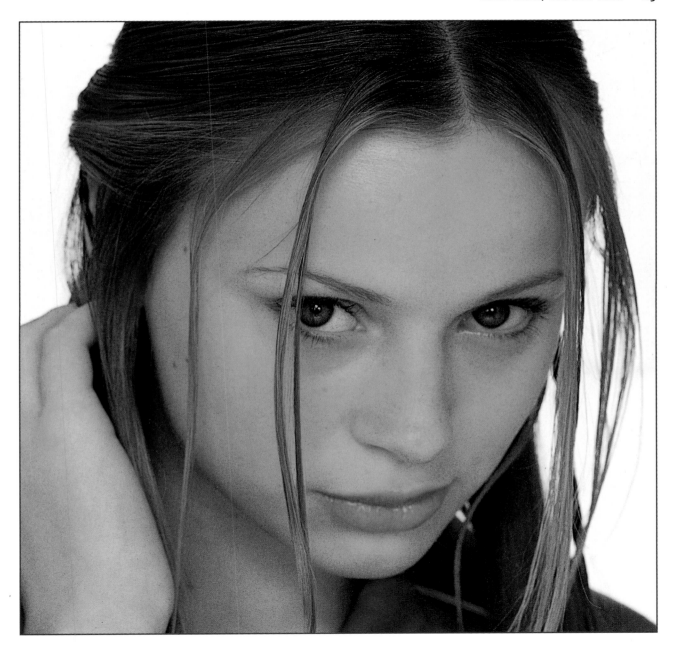

Warm Skin, Blonde Hair

Although you have a warm skin-tone, your overall look is quite delicate. This means you should opt for tawny, neutral shades of make-up, and apply them with a light touch so you enhance your basic colouring.

THIS LOOK SUITS YOU IF...

■ You have golden, warm blonde or dark blonde hair.

■ Your eyes are brown, blue, hazel or green – it will work equally well.

■ You have a warm skin-tone which can develop a light, golden tan.

■ Your skin tone and blonde hair mean your overall look is quite delicate. If so, you need to choose make-up shades that are not too intense, like those here.

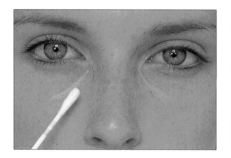

1 After applying a light, tinted moisturizer, stroke concealer onto problem areas. Blondes tend to have fine skin, often prone to surface thread veins. Cover these effectively with concealer, applied with a clean cotton bud (swab).

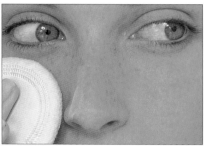

2 Dip a powder puff into loose powder and lightly press over the areas of your face that are prone to oiliness. This will absorb excess oil throughout the day, and leave your skin beautifully matte. Dust off any excess.

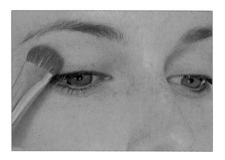

3 Sweep peach eyeshadow over your entire eyelid. It will blend with your natural skin-tone, but give a clean, wide-eyed look to your make-up.

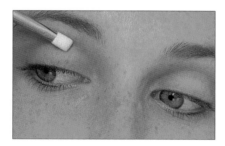

4 Use an eyeshadow brush to work a tiny amount of soft brown eyeshadow into the crease of your eyelid to create depth and definition to your eyes. Sweep it out towards the outer corner of your eyes as well.

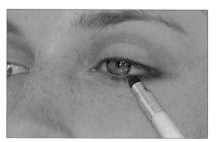

5 Still using the same brown eyeshadow, work a little underneath your lower lashes. This gives a softer effect than traditional kohl pencil or eyeliner. Finish with two coats of brown/black mascara.

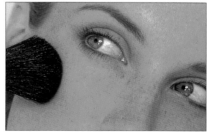

6 Apply a light shade of lipstick. Then apply your blusher, sweeping it a little at a time over your cheeks, forehead and chin. You can even dust a little over the tip of your nose!

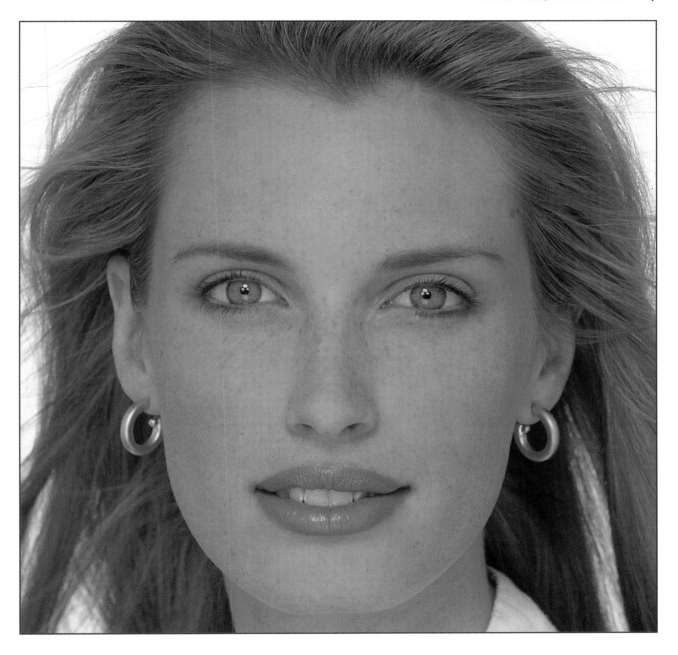

Cool Skin, Dark Hair

Pale-skinned brunettes look fabulous with strong, cool shades of cosmetics. The density of colour provides a striking contrast to ivory skin-tones, while their coolness tones in beautifully with your natural beauty.

THIS LOOK SUITS YOU IF....

■ You have medium to dark brown hair.

■ Your eyes are brown, blue, grey or green.

■ You have a cool, China doll skin-tone, that tans slowly in the sun.

Tip
To stop your mascara from clogging, wiggle the mascara wand from side to side as you pull it through your lashes.

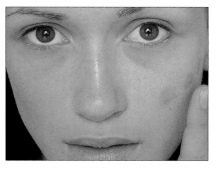

1 Apply foundation or tinted moisturizer. Whichever you use, it's likely you'll need the palest of shades. Blend in a few dots of blusher. Dust with loose powder.

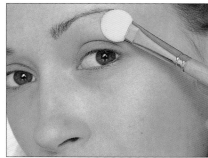

2 Smudge a cool ivory shadow over your eyelids, right up to your eyebrows. Stroke over it with a cotton bud (swab) to blend it if you find it gathers in creases.

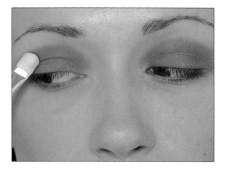

3 Add extra definition with a touch of mocha eyeshadow on your eyelids. This shade works beautifully on your cool colouring, and emphasizes the colour of your eyes.

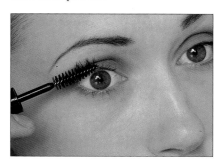

4 Now move onto your eyelashes. You need to apply two thin coats of black mascara to create a wonderful frame to your eyes.

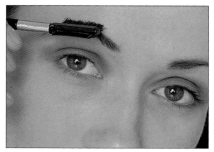

5 Slick your eyebrows into place with an eyebrow brush. If they tend to look untidy, hold them in place by spritzing the brush with a little hairspray first.

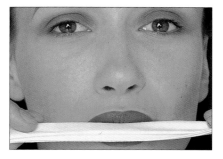

6 Choose a clear shade of berry lipstick to give your look a polished finish. Blot after one coat with a tissue, then re-apply to help a longer-lasting finish.

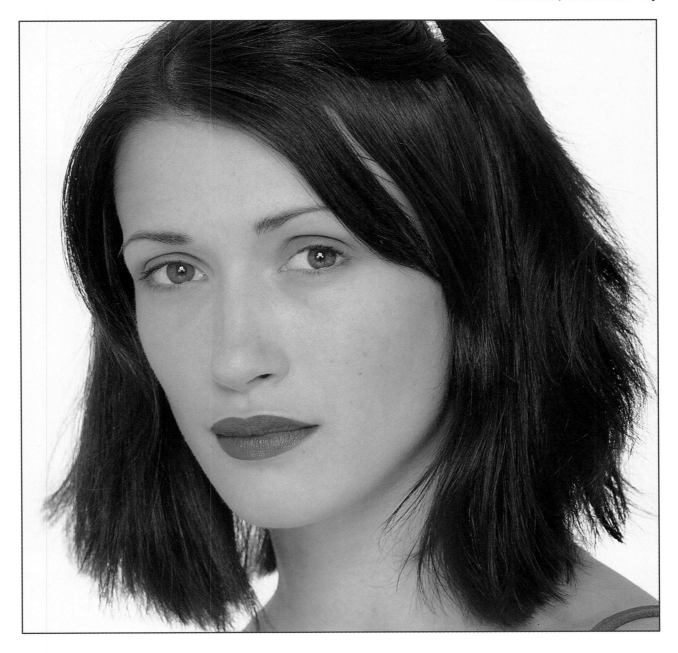

Warm Skin, Dark Hair

Your skin-tone can carry off burnished browns, warm reds and earthy shades beautifully. They'll complement your complexion and emphasize your features.

THIS LOOK SUITS YOU IF...

■ You have mid to dark brown hair.

■ Your eyes are brown, dark blue, grey, hazel or green.

■ You have a warm skin-tone that usually tans quite well. Even if it is pale in winter, your skin probably still has a yellow undertone.

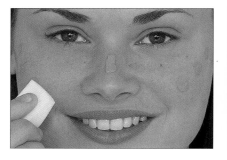

1 Dot liquid foundation onto your skin and blend in with a damp cosmetic sponge. Blend the colour into your neckline for a natural effect. Then apply concealer to any blemishes.

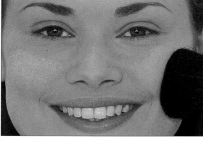

2 Pat your face with translucent loose powder, then fluff off the excess with a large, soft brush.

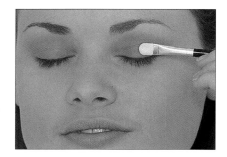

3 Use a sponge-tipped eyeshadow applicator to sweep a red-brown shadow over your entire eyelid. The advantage of the sponge over a brush is that it doesn't flick colour around.

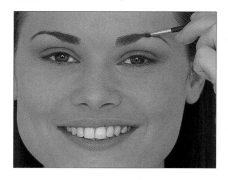

4 Your eyebrows need subtle emphasis for this look. Either pencil them in with soft strokes of brown eyebrow pencil, or use a brown eyeshadow for a softer effect. Brush and then slick the hairs in place.

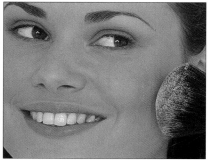

5 Opt for a warm, tawny brown shade of powder blusher, dusted over your cheeks and up towards your temples. As this colour is quite strong, you may need to tone it down a little with translucent loose powder.

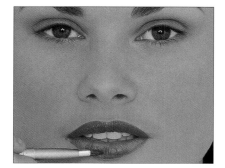

6 A fiery red lipstick balances the overall look. Use a lipbrush to ensure you fill in every tiny crease and crevice on the lip surface – this can help your lipstick colour stay put for longer as well as create a perfect finish.

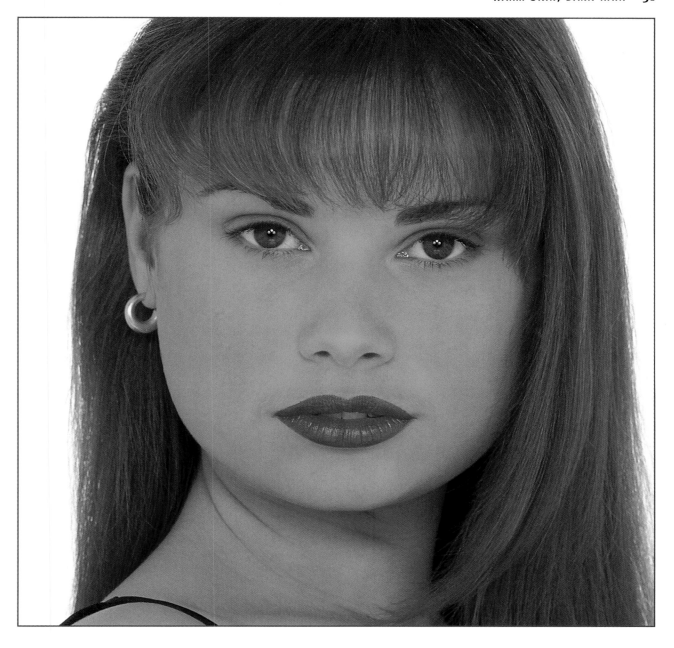

Cool Skin, Red Hair

Redheads with cool skin-tones often stick to wishy-washy colours, but you can experiment with brighter colours to contrast with your wonderful colouring. Greens give an exciting dimension to your eyes, and strong earthy shades supercharge your lips.

THIS LOOK SUITS YOU IF...

■ You have strawberry-blonde or pale red hair, even if the colour has faded.

■ Your eyes are blue, grey, hazel or green.

■ You have pale skin, ranging from ivory to a pink-toned complexion.

Tip

If you've got freckles, don't fall into the trap of trying to cover them with a dark-toned foundation. Instead, match your foundation to your skin-tone to avoid a mask-like effect.

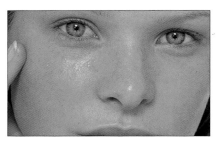

1 Apply foundation and concealer, then dot a peachy shade of blusher onto your cheekbones. Apply a little blusher at a time, and add more if you need it. Finish with loose powder.

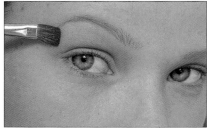

2 A neutral, peach-toned eyeshadow swept over your eyelids will emphasize your eye colour without fighting with it. Ensure you take care to work it close to your eyelashes.

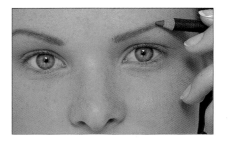

3 Opt for a very pale eyebrow pencil, in a subtle grey-brown tone. Stroke it through your eyebrows, taking care to fill any bald spots. Then soften the lines with an eyebrow brush.

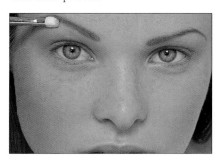

4 Brush a hint of gold, shimmery eyeshadow into the arch under your eyebrows to give your eyes an extra dimension. This is a good way to bring out gold flecks or warmth in the irises of your eyes.

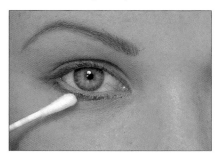

5 Work green eyeliner along your upper lashes and into the corners of your eyes as well. Smudge over the top to give a softer finish. Brush over a little translucent powder and complete with two thin coats of brown mascara.

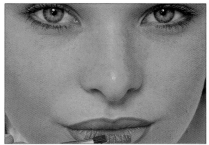

6 Burnished orange lipstick complements this look. Begin by outlining your lips with a toning lip liner to help prevent the colour from bleeding. Then use a lipbrush to fill in with the lipstick.

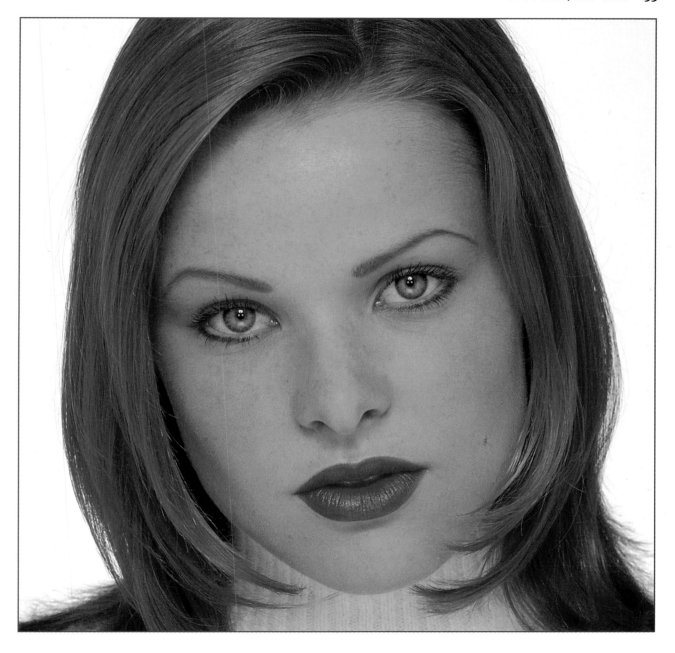

Warm Skin, Red Hair

Your vibrant Pre-Raphaelite colouring is suited to bold shades of wine, purple and brown. These deep, blue-toned colours look fabulous with your warm skin and hair tones, and can make you look truly stunning.

THIS LOOK SUITS YOU IF...

■ You have medium to dark red hair. This look may also suit brunettes who have a lot of red tones to their hair.

■ Your eyes are blue, grey, brown or green.

■ You have a medium to warm skin-tone.

■ Your skin takes on a golden colour in the summer, although you're unlikely to get a deep tan. It's quite likely that you have freckles.

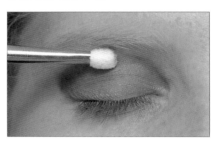

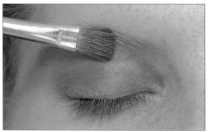

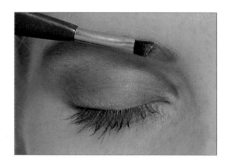

1 After applying foundation, concealer and powder, smooth a wine shade of shadow over your entire eyelid. Using a sponge-tipped eyeshadow applicator will give you more control.

2 Use a pale mauve eyeshadow over your brow bone to balance your eye make-up. Blend it into the crease, to soften any harsh edges of the wine-toned eyeshadow. Take your time at this stage, for a professional-looking finish.

3 Smudge a little eyeshadow under your lower lashes as well. Work it into the outer corners, sweeping it slightly upwards to give your eyes a lift. Then finish with two coats of brown mascara.

4 Use a soft brown eyeshadow on your eyebrows to give them subtle emphasis, using either a small brush, or a cotton bud (swab). Brush the eyebrows through afterwards with an eyebrow brush for a soft finish.

5 Choose a brown-toned blusher or bronzing powder to give your skin lots of warmth. Dust it on with a large blusher brush, blending it out towards your hairline for a natural glow. The key is to use a little at a time.

6 You can carry off a deep plum shade of lipstick, outlined with a toning lip pencil. This strong colour needs perfect application to look good, so apply two coats, blotting in between with a tissue.

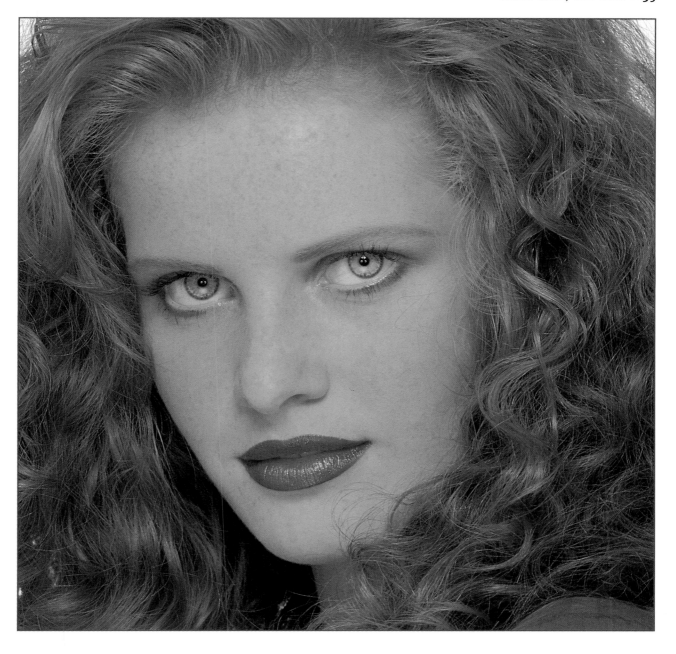

Olive Skin, Dark Hair

Your skin-tones are easy to complement with rich browns, oranges and a hint of gold or bronze. These rich shades define your features and work well on your wonderful skin-tones.

THIS LOOK SUITS YOU IF...

■ You have dark brown to black hair.

■ Your eyes are brown, hazel or green.

■ Your olive skin tans beautifully, or you have Asian or Indian colouring.

> **Tip**
> To create a perfect lip line, stretch your mouth into an "O" shape and fill in the corners with your lip pencil.

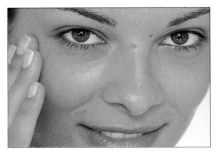

1 Even out minor skin blemishes with a tinted moisturizer, blending it in with fingertips. If you need more coverage, opt for a liquid or cream foundation. Now apply a concealer and a light dusting of face powder.

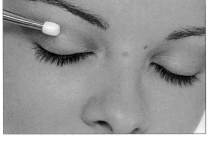

2 After sweeping a golden shade of shadow across your entire eyelid, apply a darker bronze shade into the crease and then apply some under the lower lashes. This gives a wonderfully sultry look to your eyes.

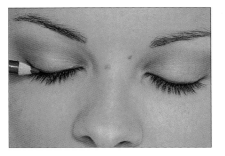

3 Take a warm brown eyeliner, and work it along your upper and lower lashes for a strong look that you can carry off beautifully. If you find the effect too harsh, lightly stroke over the top with a clean cotton bud (swab).

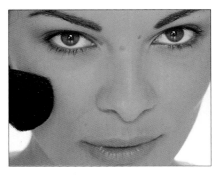

4 A peach-brown powder blusher adds a sunkissed warmth to your cheeks. Apply just a little at a time, increasing the effect as you go.

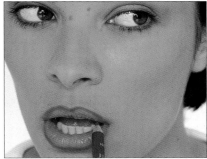

5 Outline your lips with an orange-brown lip pencil. Start at the Cupid's bow on the upper lip, and move out. Finish with the lower lip.

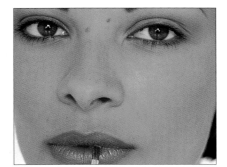

6 To complete the look, fill in with a sunny orange shade of lipstick. If you like a glamorous, glossy finish, don't blot your lips with a tissue.

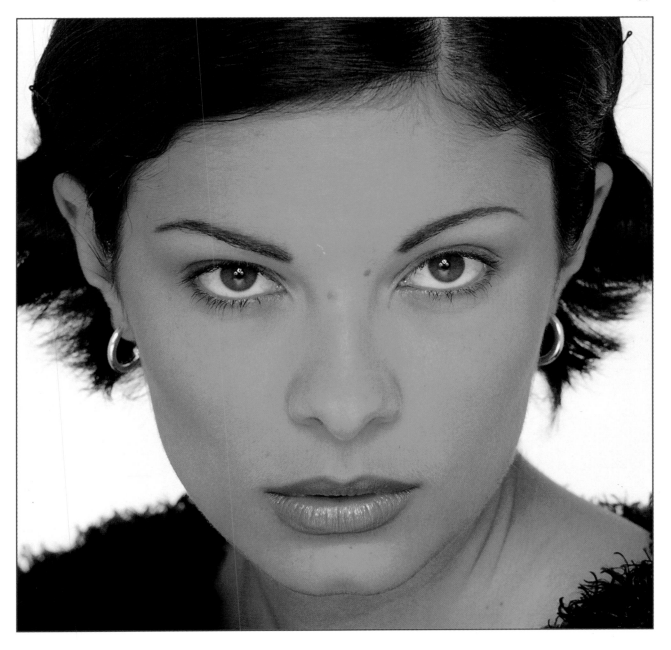

Olive Skin, Asian Colouring

Your black hair, and pale – but yellow-toned – skin are best complemented by soft, warm colours. These will define your looks and counteract any sallowness in your complexion.

THIS LOOK SUITS YOU IF...

■ You have dark brown to black hair.

■ Your eyes are hazel or brown.

■ You have a pale to medium skin-tone.

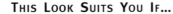

Tip
Asian eyelashes are often poker-straight and so you can really benefit from the use of eyelash curlers.

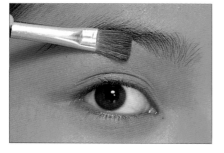

1 After applying your foundation, concealer and powder, sweep some lilac eyeshadow over your eyelid. This pale colour is a better option than using darker eyeshadows near the eyes as they have a tendency to make them look deep set, particularly as your eyelids tend to be quite small.

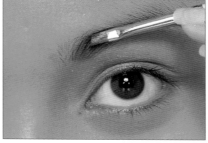

2 Lightly fill in your eyebrows with a dark brown eyeshadow or eyebrow pencil to provide a strong frame to your eyes. This will help balance the eyeliner which is going to be applied next.

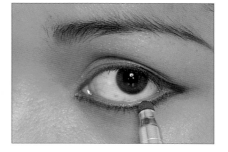

3 A lick of blue-black eyeliner will emphasize your beautifully-shaped eyes, and help correct any droopiness. Slick it along the lower lashes and into the outer corners of your eyes to create balance. To prevent the overall look from seeming too harsh, use a cotton bud (swab) to soften the eyeliner slightly.

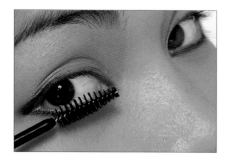

4 Place your eyelashes between the edges of a curler, and gently squeeze for a few seconds. Then apply two coats of black mascara.

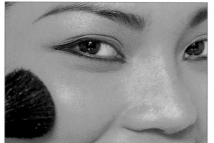

5 A warm pink blusher gives a wonderful boost to your complexion and brings out its natural glow. Dust it over the plumpest part of your cheeks.

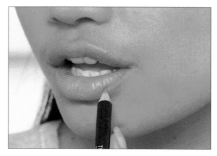

6 A baby pink lipliner and lipstick bring your lips fashionably into focus. The cool blue tone to this shade works wonderfully on your colouring.

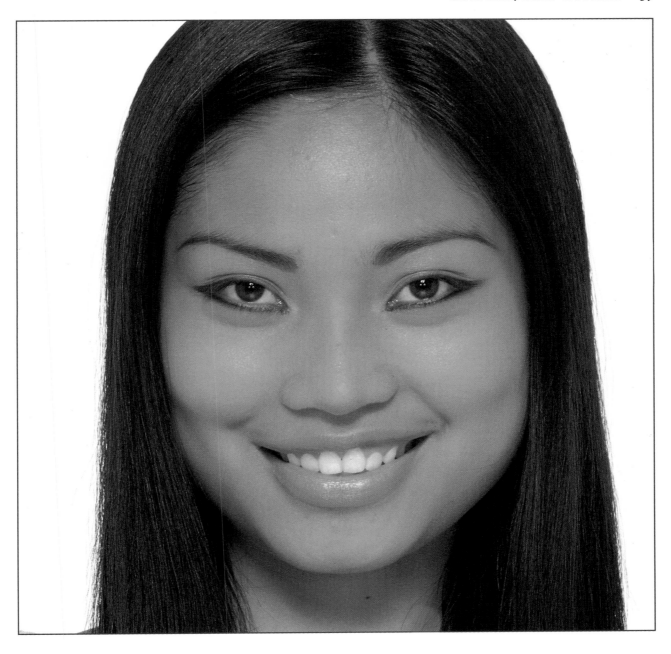

Black Hair, Pale Black Skin

Try emphasizing your looks with rich earthy shades. Your gold or red-toned skin works wonderfully with beige, brown and copper colours.

THIS LOOK SUITS YOU IF...

■ You have black hair with highlights.

■ Your have hazel or brown eyes.

■ You have black skin.

> **Tip**
> Look at cosmetic ranges especially designed for darker skins for your foundation and powder.

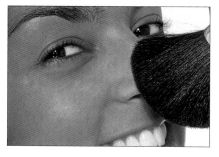

1 After applying foundation, dust on a translucent face powder, ensuring it perfectly matches your skin-tone to avoid a chalky looking complexion. Dust off the excess with a large powder brush, using downward strokes.

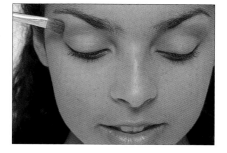

2 Use an eyeshadow brush to dust an ivory-toned eyeshadow over your entire eyelid, to create a contrast with your warm skin-tone.

3 Smudge a deep-toned brown eyeshadow into the crease of your eyelid, blending it thoroughly. Also work a little of this colour into the outer corners and underneath your lower lashes to make your eyes look really striking.

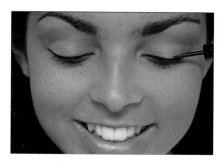

4 Sweep black liquid eyeliner along your upper lashes whilst looking down into a mirror, as this stretches creases out of your eyelid. Follow with two coats of black mascara.

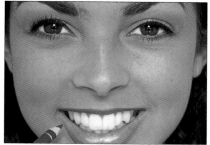

5 Use a brown lipliner pencil to outline your lips. (Use a brown eyeliner pencil if you don't have a lipliner pencil.) Blend in the line, using a cotton bud (swab) for a softer effect.

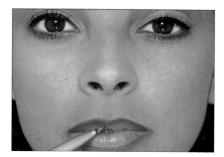

6 A neutral pink-brown lipstick gives a natural looking sheen to your lips and instantly updates your looks. Apply lipstick with a lipbrush for a perfectly even finish.

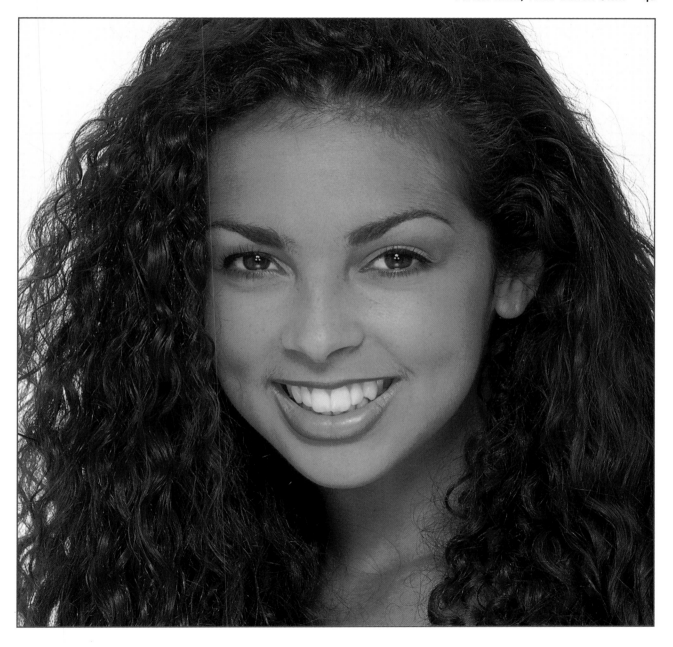

Black Hair, Deep Black Skin

You can experiment with endless colour possibilities as your dark eyes, hair and skin provide the perfect canvas on which to work. The key to success is to choose bold, deep colours as these will give your skin a wonderful glow.

THIS LOOK SUITS YOU IF...

■ You have deep black hair, even if it has flecks of grey.

■ You have dark hazel or brown eyes.

■ You have a dark black skin.

Tip
While dramatic colours suit your skin-tone and colouring perfectly, be sure to apply them with a light touch to get a fresh, up-to-date look.

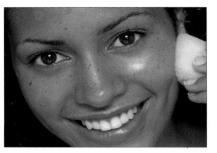

1 Choose a foundation that matches your skin-tone exactly. Apply the foundation with a damp sponge, blending it along your jaw and hairline to avoid "tidemarks" (streaks). Finally, set with a light dusting of translucent loose powder.

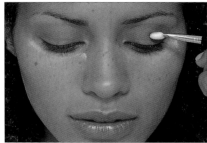

2 Next, sweep a dark blackcurrant eyeshadow over your eyelids. Dust a little loose powder under your eyes first to catch any falling specks of this dark shade, and prevent it from ruining your completed foundation.

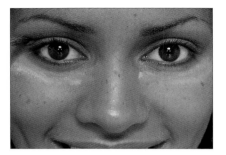

3 Apply a dark charcoal eyeshadow into the crease of your eyelid, using an eyeshadow brush. Take only a little colour at a time to the brush to prevent it from spilling on to your eyelid. If necessary, tap the brush on the back of your hand first to shake away any excess.

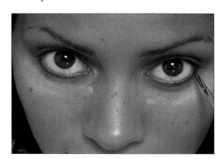

4 Use an eyeliner brush to work under your lower lashes. Hold the mirror above your eyeliner for accuracy. Finish with two coats of black mascara.

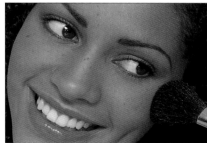

5 Choose a tawny brown shade of blusher to complement your skin. With a large brush, dust over your cheeks, working towards the hairline.

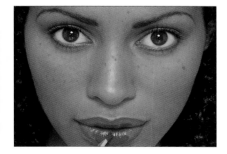

6 After outlining your lips with a toning lip pencil, fill in with a dark plum shade of lipstick, using a lipbrush.

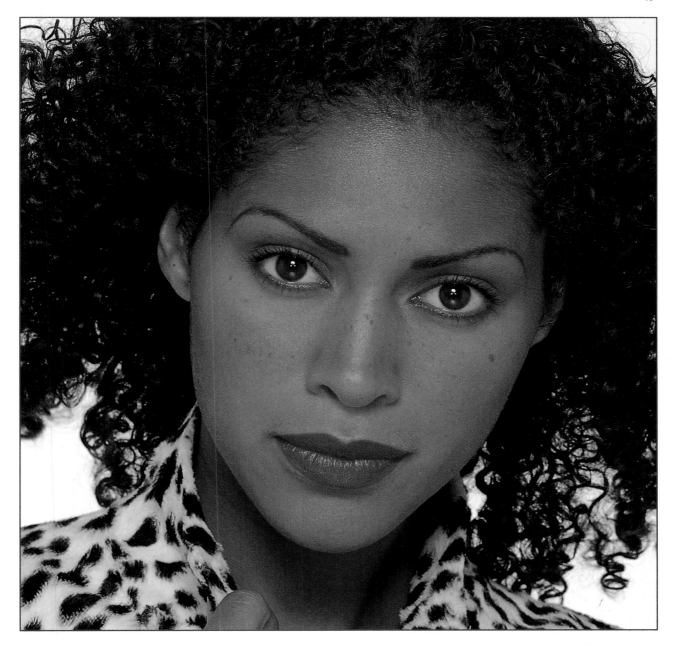

The Five-Minute Face

When you haven't got time to spare, try this quick routine for evening sophistication. The key is to choose simple looks, applied with a minimum of fuss when you're racing the clock... in other words, simple steps to a sexy look!

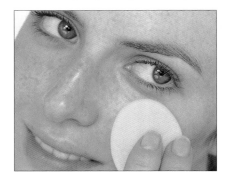

Five minutes to go...
The all-in-one foundation-powder formulations give your skin the medium coverage it needs for this look in half the time. Take it over lips and eyelids.

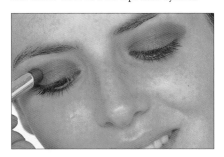

Four minutes to go...
Cream eyeshadow applied straight from the stick is quick and easy to apply. Opt for a brown shade as it'll bring out the colour of your eyes and give them a sexy, sultry finish. Slick it over your entire eyelid.

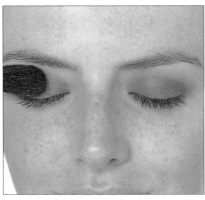

Three and a half minutes to go...
A swift way to blend in your eyeshadow is to brush over the top with translucent loose powder. This will tone down the colour and blend away any harsh edges.

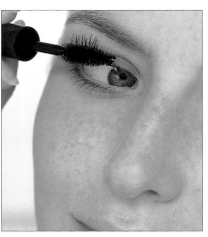

Two and a half minutes to go...
Apply a coat of mascara to your lashes, taking care to colour your lower lashes as well as your upper ones. Use the tip of the mascara wand to coat the lower lashes.

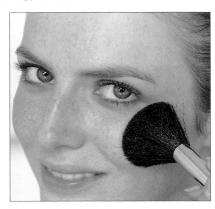

One and a half minutes to go...
A warm berry red blusher will give your skin a fabulous flush. Apply it with a blusher brush, sweeping it from your cheeks up towards your eyes.

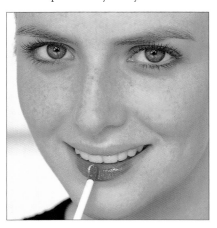

Thirty seconds to go...
Choose a berry shade of lipstick to add instant bold colour to your lips, sweeping it straight on. Cover your lower lip first, then press your lips together to transfer some of the colour onto your upper lip.

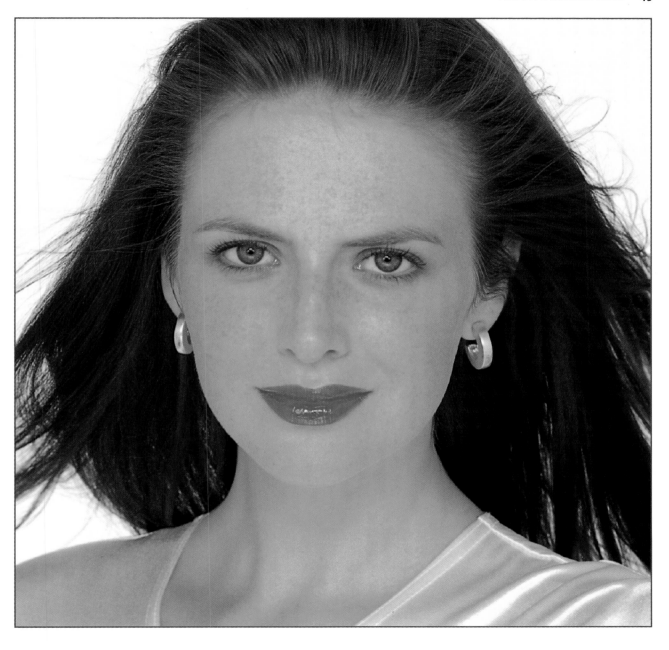

Classic Chic

Whatever your age or colouring, this simple but highly effective classic make-up look will always make a pleasing impact!

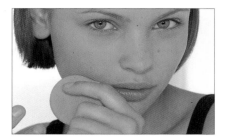

1 Apply a sheer all-in-one foundation-powder. This will give your skin the perfect coverage it needs to carry off strong lips, without clogging up your skin.

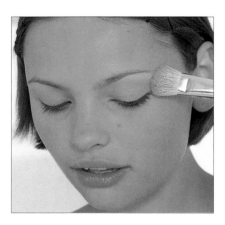

2 The eye make-up for this look is very understated. So, use eyelash curlers to open up your eyes and give them a fresh look.

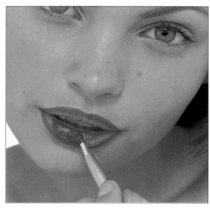

3 Sweep some pale ivory eyeshadow across your entire eyelid using a blender brush. Then complete your eyes with two thin coats of brown-black or black mascara.

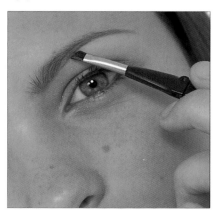

4 Well-groomed eyebrows are essential. Lightly fill in any gaps with a toning eyeshadow. This gives a softer, more natural effect than pencil.

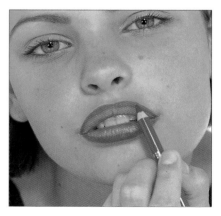

5 Your lips are the focus of this chic look. To ensure that you create a perfect outline, use a toning red lip pencil. Rest your elbow on a hard surface to prevent wobbling.

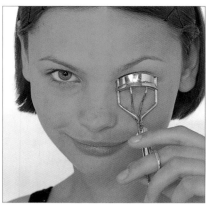

6 Use a lipbrush to fill in with a bold shade of red lipstick. Apply one coat, blot with a tissue, then reapply to help a long-lasting finish.

RED ALERT

Believe it or not, everyone can wear red lipstick. The key to success is to choose just the right shade for your colouring.

Colouring	Choose

Blonde hair, cool skin:
If you're daring enough you can wear any bright red shade. Any bold shade will look really effective and striking on you.

Blonde hair, warm skin:
Lovely pink-reds look wonderful with your colouring. They're delicate enough not to look too harsh, while the pinky undertones complement the warmth of your skin.

Dark hair, cool skin:
Rich blue wine-coloured reds look wonderful on your China doll features. The contrast of dark hair, pale skin and red lips is really stunning!

Dark hair, warm skin:
Rich brick reds and ruby jewel-like shades are very flattering to your complexion, while the intensity of colour looks great against your hair.

Red hair, cool skin:
Choose a delicate orange-red, to add a wonderful splash of colour.

Red hair, warm skin:
Warm, fiery reds with brown undertones, to complement your rich hair colour and rosy skin.

Dark hair, olive skin:
Rich red with orange undertones will flatter your skin. Go for a bold colour, as you can carry it off.

Black hair, brown skin:
Berry reds and burgundy reds look wonderful on your skin.

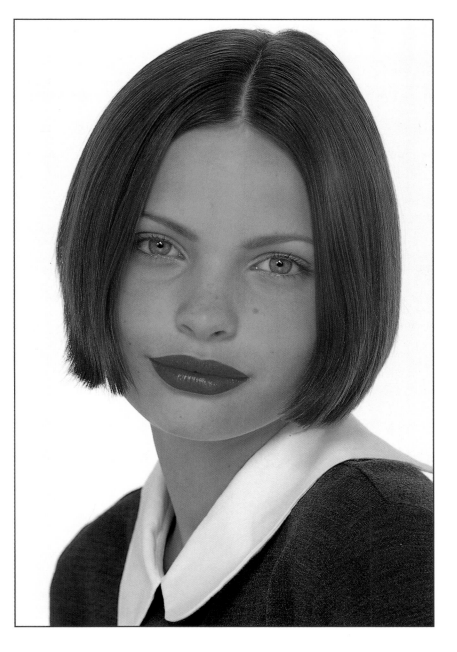

Sunkissed Country Girl

If you want a fresh, outdoor look, try this summery make-up – complete with fake freckles!

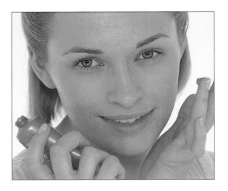

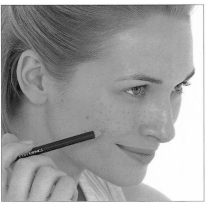

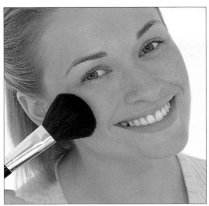

1 You need to avoid heavy foundations when you're outside, so tinted moisturizer is the perfect solution. It'll both nourish your skin and lightly cover any minor blemishes. Apply with your fingertips for ease.

2 If you already have freckles, don't try to hide them – they're perfect for a fresh-air look. If you don't have them, then fake it! Use a mid-brown eyebrow pencil, and dot freckles on the nose and cheeks. Be extra creative, and apply different sizes of freckles for a realistic look.

3 To make your faux freckles look real, soften the edges with a clean cotton bud (swab). Then dust your skin with loose powder to set them in place. A bronzing powder rather than a blusher will give your skin a sunkissed outdoor look. Dust the bronzing powder over your temples, too.

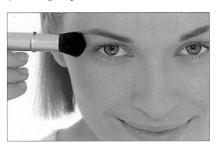

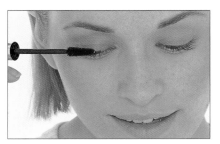

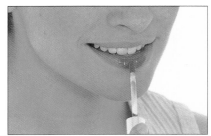

4 Swap to an eyeshadow blending brush to sweep some of the bronzing powder over your eyelids. Natural colours like brown work best for this look. Remove any harsh edges with a clean cotton bud (swab).

5 Keep mascara to a minimum. Choose a natural-looking brown or brown/black shade, and apply just one coat. The waterproof type is great for hot days and sudden downpours, but remember you'll need a waterproof eye make-up remover, too.

6 Don't overpower the look with bold lipstick. Opt for a muted brown-pink shade that's close to your natural lipcolour or use a tinted lipgloss for a natural sheen.

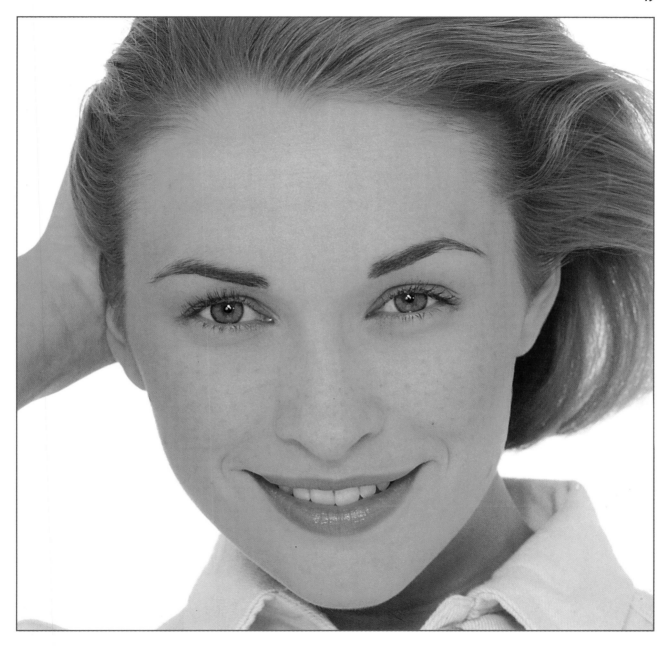

City Chic

Simple, perfectly-applied colours can help you put together a polished image. This stylish, balanced look will make you feel really confident and will leave you ready to get on with the more important things in your day!

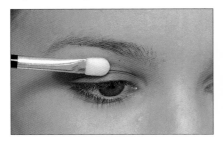

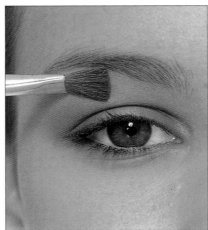

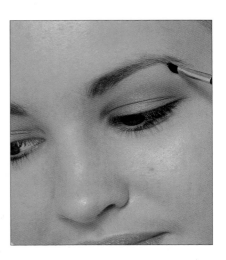

1 After applying a light foundation and dusting your skin with powder to blot out shine, sweep your eyelids with a mid-grey eyeshadow.

2 Use a beige highlighting eyeshadow over your brow bone to soften the edges of the grey shadow. Finish with two coats of mascara.

3 Brush your eyebrows with brown eyeshadow to fill in any gaps. This helps to create a strong frame to your make-up look.

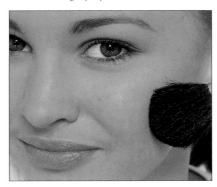

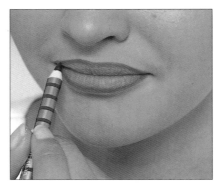

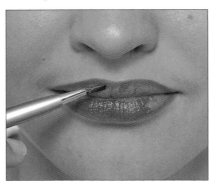

4 A soft pink shade of blusher will give your skin a rosy glow, and co-ordinate the rest of your make-up. And it will give pale work-a-day faces an immediate lift!

5 Use soft blackcurrant lipliner to outline, ensuring you take it well into the outer corners. If you create any wobbly edges, whisk over the top with a clean cotton bud (swab) dipped in a little cleansing lotion. Try again!

6 Fill in your lips with a matching shade of blackcurrant lipstick. Blot your lips with a tissue afterwards for a semi-matte finish that's perfect for a day at the office.

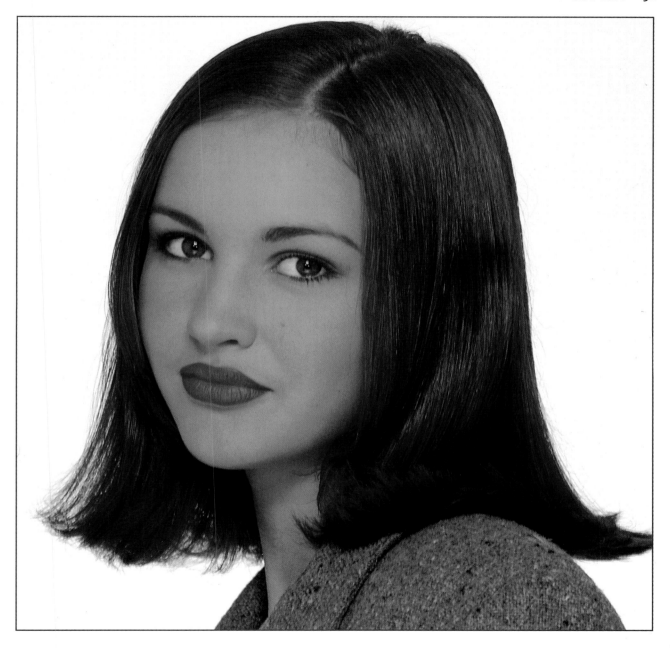

Make-Up To Look Younger!

If you haven't changed your make-up in years, it's a fair bet you're not making the most of your looks. Wearing out-of-fashion make-up is a sure way to add years to your appearance. Our simple make-up rules will help you break out of a beauty rut.

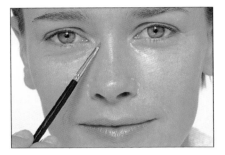

Simple steps to perfect skin

A dull, lifeless skin-tone can make you look, and feel, drab. The great news is, there are now foundations and concealers on the market specially designed to deal with this problem. The formulations contain light-reflective particles, and these bounce light away from your skin. This gives your skin the illusion of added vitality, and helps disguise problem areas such as fine lines and under-eye shadows.

And the good news is that these light-reflective products are not just limited to expensive beauty counters — many more price-conscious companies are now offering them too.

Apply foundation with a damp sponge, blending away harsh edges. This is the stage to apply concealer, dotting it on to under-eye shadows, blemishes and thread veins with a brush. Apply a little at a time, and blend it in thoroughly.

Before you start

Avoid extremes of fashion and bright colours when you're over 40. While younger skins can just about get away with garish make-up, it'll simply emphasize fine lines and wrinkles on most women. Concentrate instead on flattering your looks with subtle colours. So, throw away those traffic-stopping blue eyeshadows and neon lipsticks!

If you haven't a clue where to start, make an appointment for a free makeover at a local beauty counter. This way you'll be able to see which shades suit you before you launch out and buy.

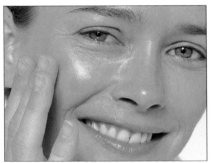

Add a youthful glow with blusher

Forget about adding colour to your skin with foundation — you'll be left with a mask effect and "tidemarks" (streaks) on your jawline. Instead, recreate a youthful bloom with a light touch of blusher. Remember though, to use half as much blusher and twice as much blending as you originally think! The cream variety of blusher is a good one to try, because it will give your skin a soft glow. Dot the blusher onto your skin, and blend with your fingertips.

Lightly set your foundation and blusher with translucent powder. A common mistake among many women is to be heavy-handed with face powder. Applying too much can make it settle into fine lines and wrinkles on your face and emphasize them. Aim for a light touch, which will just blot out shine and set your make-up.

The best way to apply powder is only to blot the areas that need it, then brush away the excess with a large powder brush, stroking the brush downwards to prevent tiny particles catching in the fine hairs on your face.

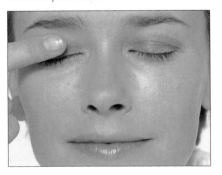

Be subtle with eyeshadow

Many women never perfect the technique of applying eyeshadow. Thankfully, now there's a type of eyeshadow formulation that is a cinch to apply — cream-to-powder eyeshadow. It applies as a smooth cream, and dries quickly to a super-soft powder finish. Opt for a subtle shade, such as mid-brown, grey or taupe.

A good tip if your eyes look rather droopy is to blend eyeshadow upwards and outwards at the outer corners. Always remember to blend it in well.

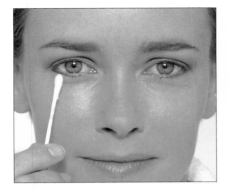

Give eyeliners a miss

Harsh lines of colour close to your eyes can be hard and unflattering. You'll emphasize your eyes much better if you smudge a little neutral-toned powder eyeshadow under your lower lashes with a clean cotton bud (swab).

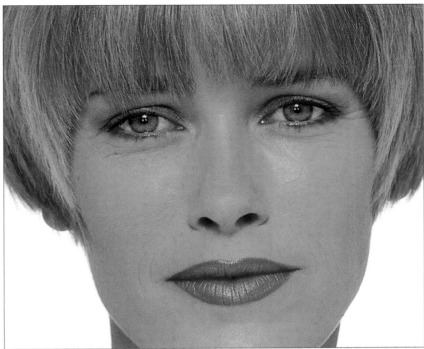

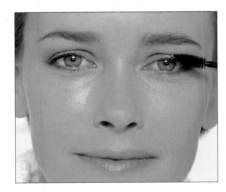

Check your mascara colour

Most women's colouring fades slightly over the years. This means that the black mascara you're used to wearing can now look too obvious and harsh. So, try switching to a lighter shade for a more flattering effect. Apply two thin coats, allowing time for the first to dry thoroughly before you apply the second one.

Recreate your lip line

If your lip line has started to fade and your lipstick tends to "bleed" into the lines around your mouth, try using a toning lipliner before you apply lipstick. Check it's firm enough to give a precise line, yet soft enough not to drag your skin. Apply by outlining your top lip first, working from the Cupid's bow outwards to each corner. Then outline your lower lip. Next dust your lips with loose powder to set the lipliner.

Finally, fill in your outline with a moisturizing lipstick. This will also help give a glossy shine to your lips which makes them look fuller. Apply with a lipbrush, blot with a tissue, then reapply for a longer-lasting finish.

Above: Break out of a beauty rut and achieve a youthful new look!

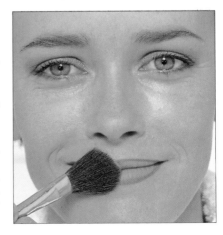

Go For Glamour!

If there's one time you want to make a special effort with your make-up and pull out all the stops, it's a big night out!

We'll show you how to create this stunning look, which combines a mixture of dark and light tones.

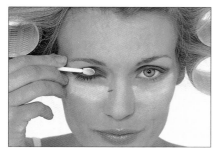

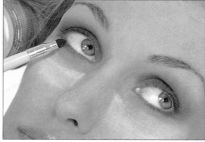

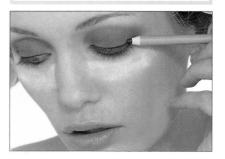

1 After applying your foundation, concealer and powder, you're ready to work on your eye make-up. Sweep a smoky dark brown eyeshadow over your entire eyelid and blend it carefully into the crease. A sponge applicator is easier to use than a brush, but sweep a line of loose powder under your eyes to catch any falling specks of dark shadow.

2 Apply a little of the same shade of eyeshadow under your lower lashes to accentuate the shape of your eyes. This will give a balanced look to your eye make-up and provide a smooth base on which to apply your eyeliner at the next stage. The emphasis for this look is on glamour and impact!

3 Whereas black eyeliner is usually too severe for harsh daylight, it's perfect for this look, which is designed to be seen in softer, sexier light! Using a pencil, carefully draw a fine line above and below your eyelashes. If you find it hard to create a steady hand, try drawing a series of tiny dots, then blend them together with a clean cotton bud (swab).

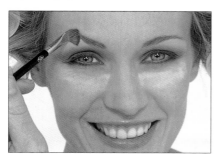

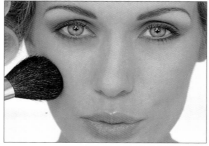

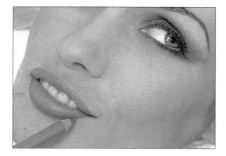

4 To contrast the dark look on your eyelids, sweep a pearlized ivory shadow over your brow bones. Build up the effect gradually. Complete the look with two coats of black mascara.

5 Use tawny blushes or a bronzing powder for this look – they won't compete with the rest of your make-up. Sweep it over your cheekbones and blend away the edges into your hairline.

6 Keeping the lips neutral gives this look its real impact and updates it. Opt for a pinkish-beige shade of lip pencil and smudge it over your entire mouth for a matte, understated effect.

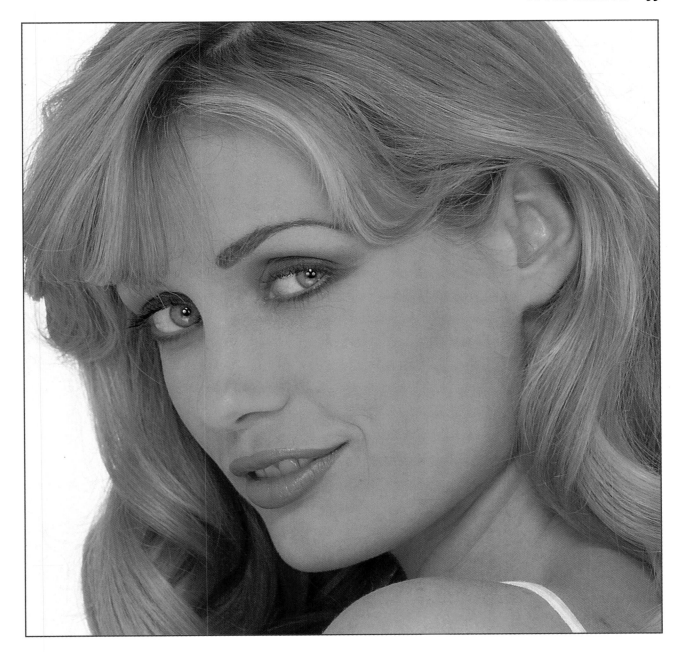

20 Problem Solvers

Whether you have made a beauty mistake, have run out of a vital product or are simply stuck for inspiration on how to make the most of your looks, the following problem solvers are just what you need!

Problem 1

Polish remover has run out

If you want to re-paint your nails, but have run out of remover, try coating one nail at a time with a clear base coat. Leave to dry for a few seconds, then press a tissue over the nail and remove it at once – the base coat and coloured polish will come off in one quick move.

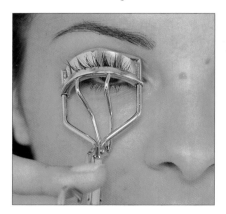

Problem 2

Poker-straight lashes

Do invest in a set of eyelash curlers, as they really make a difference to the way your eyes look. Gently squeeze your lashes between their cushioned pad before applying mascara or you'll risk breaking off the hairs. Curling your lashes makes them look thicker than usual and helps to open up the eyes.

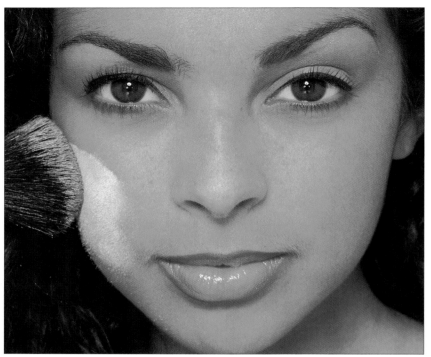

Problem 3

Patchy powder

Provided you apply your powder with a light touch to freshly moisturized skin or on top of foundation that's applied with a clean sponge, it should look perfect. Check your powder is matched closely to your natural skin-tone. So, try dusting a sample of powder onto your skin in natural daylight before buying.

Problem 4

Stained nails

Stained nails are usually caused by wearing dark-coloured nail polish without using a protective clear base coat. Try switching to paler coloured polishes, as these contain lower levels of pigment that are less likely to stain your nails, and use a clear base coat underneath.

Problem 5

Flaky mascara

This usually means the mascara is old and the oils that keep it creamy have dried out. Try not to pump air into the dispenser – go gently when replacing the cap – and replace your mascara every few months. If mascara flakes on your lashes, remove it and make a clean start.

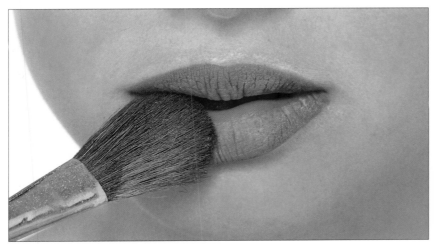

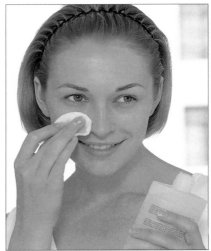

Problem 6
Melting lipstick
If you're out and about and your lipstick is starting to move in the heat, then dust over the top with a little loose powder. This will give it a slightly drier texture, to help it stay put for longer. A little loose powder will also create a lovely matte finish.

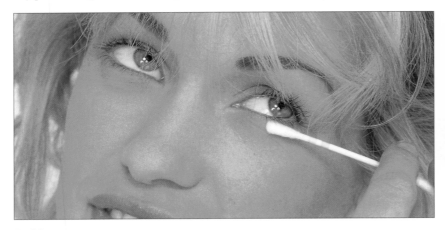

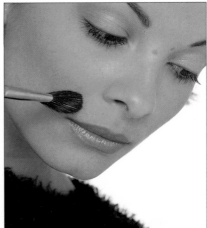

Problem 7
Smudged eyeliner
Tidy up the under-eye area by dipping a cotton bud (swab) into some eye make-up remover. Whisk it over the problem area to remove smudges, then re-powder. In future, remember to run a little loose powder over eyeliner to combat smudging.

Problem 8
A blemish appears
Start by calming down the blemish by dabbing it with a gentle astringent. Apply a concealer directly onto the blemish or spot, and tidy up the edges with a clean cotton bud (swab). Set in place with a light dusting of loose powder.

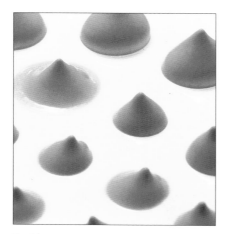

Problem 9
Red-toned skin or embarrassing blushes
A red skin colour can be toned down by smoothing your skin with a specialized green-tinted foundation. Apply with a light touch, just to the areas that really need it. The green pigment in the cream has the effect of cancelling out the red in your skin.

However, to avoid a ghostly glow, you'll need to apply a light coating of your ordinary foundation on top and then set with a dusting of loose powder. This tip is also good for covering the occasional angry spot or blemish.

Problem 10
Flaky lips
If your lips are flaky you'll find it difficult to create a smooth lipstick finish. Slick your lips with petroleum jelly, and leave for 10 minutes to give it time to soften hard flakes of skin. Then cover your index finger with a damp flannel and gently massage your lips. This will remove the petroleum jelly and the flakes of dead skin at the same time.

Problem 11
Bleeding lipstick
Use lipliner to help prevent your lipstick from bleeding into the fine lines around your mouth. Trace the lip outline, then apply lip colour with a brush. Choose a drier textured matte lipstick as they're less prone to bleeding. Also, lightly powder over and around your lips before you start.

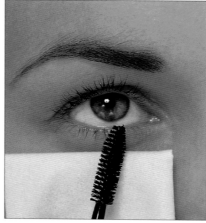

Problem 12
Smudged mascara
If your mascara always seems to run onto your skin, leaving you with "panda eyes", first check that you are using a water-proof variety. Try holding a piece of tissue just underneath your lower lashes while you're applying your mascara to prevent it from getting as far as your skin in the first place.

Alternatively, dip a cotton bud (swab) in eye make-up remover for fast touch-ups before the mascara has a moment to dry on your skin.

To remove excess mascara, place a tissue between your upper and lower lashes and blink two or three times.

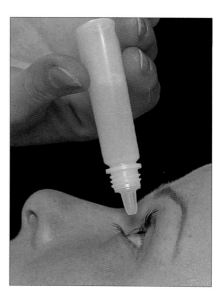

Problem 13
Bloodshot eyes
Red eyes are caused by the swelling of the tiny blood vessels on the eye surface, which can be caused by lack of sleep, excessive time in front of a computer, a smoky atmosphere or an infection. If it's a continual problem, consult your doctor, or ask your optician for an eyesight examination to ensure there's nothing to worry about.

On a temporary basis, you can use eye drops to bring a fresh sparkle back to your eyes.

Problem 14
Tidemarks of foundation
If you find obvious edges to your foundation on your chin, jawline or hairline, blend them away with a damp cosmetic sponge. Do this in natural daylight so you can check the finished effect. Powder as usual afterwards.

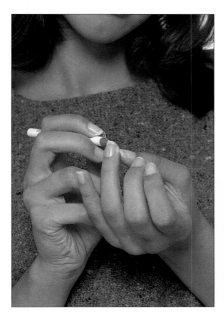

Problem 15
Unhealthy-looking nails

Sometimes, however strong your nails are, their overall effect can be spoilt by yellowing tips. However, you can immediately improve them by running a white manicure pencil underneath the free edges of nail to give them a cleaner appearance. Combine with a coat of clear polish for a fresh, natural nail look.

Problem 16
Yellow teeth

First of all, consult your dentist or dental hygienist for regular check-ups and thorough cleaning. Take heart: yellow teeth tend to be stronger than their whiter counterparts! To make them look whiter, avoid coral or brown-based lipsticks — clear pink or red shades will make your teeth look much whiter in comparison.

Problem 17
Droopy eyes

To help lift the appearance of droopy eyes, sweep a light-toned eyeshadow all over your eyelid. Then apply a little eyeshadow with a clean cotton bud (swab) under your eyes, sweeping it slightly upwards. Apply extra coats of mascara on the lashes just above the iris of the eye to draw attention to the centre of your eye rather than the outer corners.

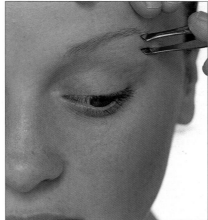

Problem 18
Straggly eyebrows

Tidy them with regular tweezing sessions. The ideal time is after a bath, when your pores will be open from the heat. Before bedtime is also a great idea, so you don't have to face the day with reddened skin!

Quickly brush your brows into place, so you can see the natural shape. Then pluck one hair at a time, in the direction of growth. First remove the hairs between your brows, and then tweeze any stray hairs at the outer sides. As a general rule, don't pluck above the eyebrow area.

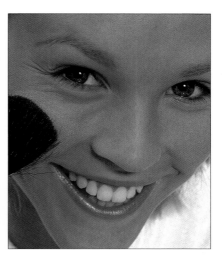

Problem 19
Over-applied blusher

If you've forgotten the golden rule about building up your blusher slowly and gradually, you may need to tone down an over-enthusiastic application of colour. The quickest and easiest way is to dust a little loose powder over the top of the problem area until you've reached a depth of blusher shade that you're happy with.

Problem 20
Over-plucked eyebrows

Choose a natural-looking brown eyeshadow. Then apply it lightly and evenly with a firm-bristled eyebrow brush, using short sharp strokes across the brow. As the hairs that grow back are often unruly, a light coat of clear mascara can be applied to help keep them in place.

Try to ignore the periodic fashions for highly plucked eyebrows. The fashions don't last for long — but eyebrows can take ages to grow back!

Hands Up to Beautiful Nails

Alittle manual labour is all it takes to have hands to be proud of – rather than ones you want to hide!

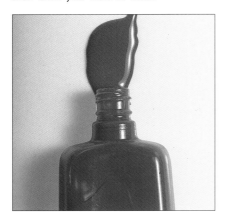

Above: Give your nails a splash of colour for instant glamour.

Filing know how

Keep your nails slightly square or oval – not pointed – to prevent them from breaking. Filing low into the corners and sides can weaken nails. File gently in one long stroke, from the side to the centre of the nail. The classic length that suits most hands is just over the fingertip.

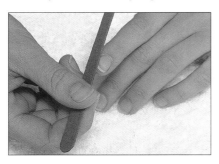

Condition-plus

Good-looking nails need to be in condition. Smooth your nails every evening with a nourishing oil or conditioning cream. This helps seal moisture into your nails to prevent flaking and splitting.

Cuticle care

Go carefully with tough or overgrown cuticles. Soak your nails in warm, soapy water to soften the cuticles. Then smooth them with a little cuticle softening cream or gel, before gently pushing them back with a manicure hoof stick or clean cotton bud (swab). You can then gently scrub away the flakes of dead skin that are still clinging to the nail bed.

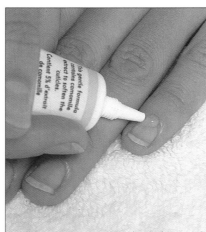

Above: Most manicurists advise against cutting cuticles with scissors – do use the proper cream.

Left: Use an emery board rather than a metal file.

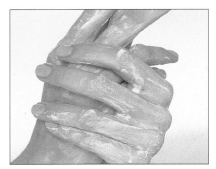

TOP 10 NAIL TIPS

1 If you have very soft nails, file them while the polish is still on.

2 Apply hand cream every time you wash your hands.

3 Wear rubber gloves when doing the washing-up.

4 If you have very weak nails, try painting base coat and nail polish under the tips.

5 Dry wet nail polish with a cold jet of air from your hairdryer.

6 Leave a tiny polish-free gap at the base of the nail where the cuticle meets the nail – this is where the new nail cells are growing.

7 If you're planning to do some gardening or messy work, drag your nails over a bar of soap. The undersides of your nails will fill up with soap, which means dirt won't be able to get in.

8 Clean ink and stains from your fingertips by using a toothbrush and toothpaste on the affected areas.

9 Hide cracked or chipped nails under stick-on false ones – only for a temporary solution!

10 Use a cotton bud (swab) with a pointed end to clean under your nails – it's gentler than scrubbing with a nail brush.

COLOUR CODING

■ If you have long, elegant fingers, you can carry off any shade of polish, including the dramatic deep reds, russets and burgundies.

■ Short nails look their best with pale or beige-toned polish.

■ Pale colours also suit broad nails. However, you can make them look slightly narrower by leaving a little space on the sides of each nail unpainted.

■ If you love nude, barely-there shades for the daytime, but prefer something more exotic at night, try a pale pearlized polish – the shimmer will be caught by the evening light.

■ Coral polish and pearlized formulations work wonderfully against a tanned skin.

■ If you find strong colours too bold on your hands, try painting your toenails instead. A glimpse of wonderful colour in open-toed shoes or on bare feet can look very sophisticated. You can create our model look by mixing a little dark red and black nail polish together before applying.

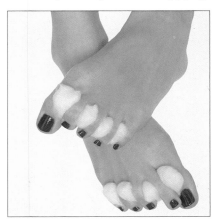

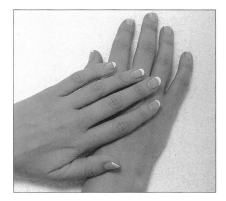

Above: French polish your nails to make them look clean and fresh.

POLISH UP YOUR FRENCH!

When it comes to nail trends, there's one look that never goes out of fashion, and that's the French manicure. It leaves your nails looking clean, fresh and healthy – and matches any make-up you happen to be wearing.

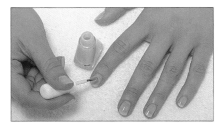

1 The basis of the French manicure is two coats of pale pink polish. Copy the professionals and do it in three strokes – one down the middle and one on each side. Apply two coats, giving each one plenty of time to dry. To turn a French manicure into an "American manicure", switch the pink polish for a beige one.

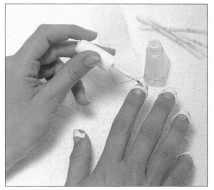

2 Now it's time to paint the tips of your nails with a white polish. If you find it difficult to paint them freehand, try using the stick-on nail guards that come with many French manicure sets. Rest your hands on a firm surface to keep them steady.

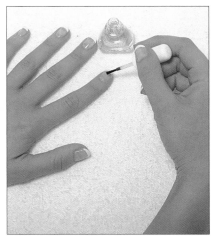

3 Once the white tips of your nails are dry, paint on a clear top coat of polish to seal in the colour and create a chip-resistant finish.

50 Fast, Effective Beauty Tips

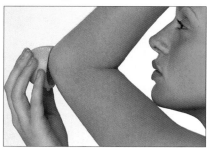

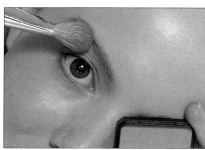

1 Brighten grey elbows by rubbing them with half a fresh lemon – it has a natural bleaching effect. Moisturize the skin afterwards to counteract the drying effects of the juice.

2 Turn foundation into tinted moisturizer by mixing a few drops of it with a little moisturizer on the back of your hand before applying. It's the perfect blend for summer.

3 Carry a spray of mineral water in your handbag to freshen up foundation while you're out and about.

4 Sleeping on your back helps prevent wrinkles, according to recent research. It's certainly worth a try!

5 Dunk feet into a bowl containing warm water and 4 tablespoons of Epsom salts to help ease swollen ankles.

6 If you have very soft nails, file them while the polish is still on to prevent them from cracking.

7 If you find eyebrow tweezing painful, hold an ice cube over the area first to numb the area before you start.

8 Warm up your looks by dusting a little blusher over your temples, chin and the tip of your nose as well as your cheeks.

9 Sweep a little loose powder under your eyes when applying dark shades of eye-shadow to catch any falling specks and prevent them from staining your skin.

10 Make your lips look larger by wearing a bright, light lipstick. Or make them appear smaller by wearing dark or more muted colours.

11 Soak nails in a bowl of olive oil once a week to strengthen them.

12 Keep your smile looking its best by changing your toothbrush as soon as the bristles begin to splay. This means at least every three months. You should brush for at least two minutes, both morning and night.

13 If you don't have a specialized contouring product for your cheeks, simply use an ordinary face powder a couple of shades darker than your usual one to slim round cheeks.

14 Add a drop of witch hazel – available in all good pharmacies – to turn ordinary foundation into a medicated one – it'll work wonders on oily skin or skin which is prone to blemishes.

15 Mascara your lashes before applying false ones to help them stick properly.

16 If you look tired, blend a little concealer just away from the outer corner of your eye – it makes you look as though you had a good night's sleep!

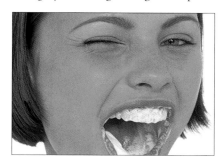

17 Go lightly with powder on wrinkles around the eyes – too much will settle into them and emphasize them.

18 If you haven't got time for a full make-up, but want to look great, paint on a bright red lipstick – it's a happy, glamorous colour which immediately brightens your face.

19 When plucking your eyebrows, coat the hairs you want to remove with concealer – it'll help you visualize exactly the shape of brow you're after.

20 Never apply your make-up before blow-drying your hair – the heat from the dryer can make you perspire and cause your make-up to smudge.

21 The colour of powder eyeshadow can be made to look more intense by dipping your eyeshadow brush in water first.

22 Keep lashes smooth and supple by brushing them with petroleum jelly before going to bed at night, or use to emphasize natural-looking lashes.

23 Apply cream blusher in light downward movements, to prevent it from creasing in specks of colour from catching in the fine hairs on your face.

24 If mascara tends to clog on your lower lashes, try using a small thin brush to paint colour on to individual lashes.

25 Make sure you give moisturizer time to sink in before you start applying your make-up – it'll help your make-up go on more easily.

26 For eyes that really sparkle, try outlining them just inside your eyelashes with a soft white cosmetic pencil.

27 Lip gloss can look sophisticated if you just apply a dot in the centre of your lower lip.

28 Hide cracked or chipped nails under stick-on false ones.

29 If your eyeliner is too hard and drags your skin, hold it next to a light bulb for a few seconds before applying.

30 If you find your lashes clog with mascara, try rolling the brush in a tissue first to blot off the excess, leaving a light, manageable film on the bristles.

31 If you're unsure where to apply blusher, gently pinch your cheeks. If you like the effect, apply blusher in the same area – it'll look wonderfully natural.

32 To prevent lipstick from getting on your teeth, try this tip: after putting it on, put your finger in your mouth, purse your lips and pull it out.

33 Women who wear glasses need to take special advice on make-up. If you're near-sighted, your glasses will make your eyes look smaller. So, opt for brighter,

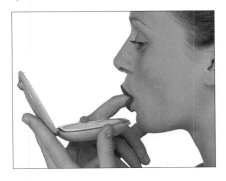

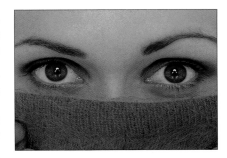

bolder shadows and lots of mascara to ensure they don't disappear. If you're far-sighted, your lenses will make your eyes look bigger and your eye make-up more prominent. So, opt for more muted colours that won't seem so obvious.

34 For a long-lasting blush on sunny days or hot nights, apply both cream and powder blusher. Apply the cream formulation first, set with translucent powder then dust with a little powder blush.

35 Let your nails breathe by leaving a tiny gap at the base of the nail where the cuticle meets the nail – this is where the new nail cells are growing.

36 A little foundation lightly rubbed through your eyebrows and brushed through with an old toothbrush will instantly lighten them.

37 Coloured mascara can look super-effective if applied with a light hand. Start by coating your lashes with two coats of black mascara. Once the lashes are dry, slick a coloured mascara – try blue, violet or green – onto the underside of your upper lashes. Each time you blink your eyelashes will reveal a dash of colour.

38 If you use hypo-allergenic make-up for sensitive skin, remember to choose hypo-allergenic nail polish, too – you constantly touch your face with your hands and can easily trigger a reaction.

39 Make over-prominent eyes appear smaller by applying a wide coat of liquid liner. The thicker the line the smaller your eyes will look.

40 Calm down an angry red blemish by holding an ice cube over it for a few seconds and then apply your usual medicated concealer.

41 If you've run out of loose powder, use a light dusting of unperfumed talcum powder instead.

42 Use a little green eyeshadow on red eyelids to mask the ruddiness.

43 If you've run out of liquid eyeliner, dip a thin brush into your mascara and apply in the same way. It works perfectly.

44 You can dry nail polish quickly by blasting nails with a cold jet of air from your hairdryer.

45 Use a toothpick or dental floss regularly to clean between your teeth, and make sure you visit the dentist every 6 months to avoid serious problems.

46 Apply foundation-powder with a damp sponge for a thicker, more opaque coverage. Applied with a dry sponge, the result will be sheerer.

47 Run your freshly sharpened eyeliner pencil across a tissue before use. This will round off any sharp edges and remove small particles of wood.

48 If you have hard-to-cover under-eye shadows, cover them with a light coat of blue cream eyeshadow before using your ordinary concealer. It really works.

49 Get together with a friend and make each other up – it's amazing how other people picture you – and it's a great way to find yourself a new look.

50 Remove excess mascara by placing a folded paper tissue between your upper and lower lashes and then blinking two or three times.

Index

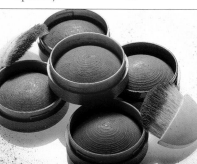